Conquering Cancer...

By Susan Gorkosky and
John Lubecki, D.C.

info@juicingforcancer.com
www.juicingforcancer.com
www.lubecki-chiropractic.com

Conquering Cancer...
By Susan Gorkosky and John Lubecki, D.C.

Published by:
Susan Gorkosky and John Lubecki, D.C.
California, USA

Cover art designed by: Collene Irish

Copyright © 2011 by Susan Gorkosky and John Lubecki, D.C.:
First Edition, 2011

ISBN 9780983890607

Published in the United States of America

DEDICATION

This book is dedicated to Sally Cole, my sister, my best friend, mentor and caregiver. Her perspective on life made me laugh when I wanted to cry, gave me strength when I felt like quitting, gave me perspective when I thought things like "all foods are toxic". She walked with me, slept with me when I was scared, she cooked for me, drove me to doctors' appointments (tons of them), never judged me when I tried treatment after treatment and forgave me for all the times when I couldn't be as kind as I needed to be. She gave me the tough love when I needed it, but never forgot my frailty, mental and physical. She is always funny and giving. She could be as tough as John Wayne and soft as Marilyn Monroe that is her fabulous winning combo.

My hero award goes to Dr. John Lubecki. He is my tireless crusader for good health. In his 40+years career he has helped thousands of people restore themselves to good health. Thank you so much for helping me heal myself.

Thank you both for your diligence and for giving me the tools that I needed to beat this cancer and for giving me "Hope and Inspiration" when around me I only saw "Fear and Desperation".

Susan Gorkosky

TABLE OF CONTENTS

INTRODUCTION

DISCLAIMER

INTRODUCTION

Today it is absolutely impossible for medical doctors to keep up with all the new drugs, new treatments, and new equipment available in orthodox medicine, much less, alternative treatments. Our medical system has become compartmentalized. You see a specialist for just about everything. Like the spokes on a wheel each doctor knows one system in your body, your total body health is just what's written in your file: your extensive tests, your diagnosis.

For example, I just received my ten year colonoscopy. My gastroenterologist (specialist) told me that I was going to see a surgeon in the following month. He showed me in his computer file where it said I had something wrong in my colon. I said "no I don't, this is a routine examination" to which he replied "no you need surgery it's right here in your file".

The colonoscopy was just perfect, no problems at all. As I left he reminded me of my appointment with the surgeon. He believed what my computer file said not me. What is wrong with this picture?

At this moment you need to become your own "Healthcare Boss". You need to ask the right questions, research drugs and their side effects, become your own healthcare advocate.

The first time you go to your general practitioner they listen to you. They then try to isolate a specific problem and get you on the "Medical Wheel" of specialists. They do listen that first time, but rarely do they explain much. The doctor will either prescribe a drug that will cut off the "warning light" (symptom) in your body or send you for a series of tests to decide what specialist you need.

Symptoms like pain, headache, fever, are the body's warning lights that something is not right in your body. If you took your car to a mechanic because the oil light on your dashboard was on you wouldn't expect him to operate on your dashboard. Many drugs prescribed to us just cut off the warning signals of the body. Drugs can be very harmful to our bodies and their side effects can be devastating.

Fifteen years ago I went to my doctor and said I was having trouble sleeping so she prescribed Klonopin (generic form Clonazepam). I slept like a baby, I loved it. When I was diagnosed with my brain cancer I decided to go off of all my prescription drugs. I was taking Vicodin for pain, Valium for depression, Soma as a muscle relaxer and Clonazepan for sleep. I was able to get off of the Vicodin and Soma with limited side effects or so I think. But the Valium was like coming off of some street drug... sweating, fatigue, and shaking. The Clonazepan I found out was actually a very old drug that was an "anti-seizure" drug. One of the side effects was sleepiness so it was prescribed to me for sleep. When I tried to go off it "cold turkey" I started having seizures. I looked it up on the internet and sure enough the side effects included "causes seizures." Unfortunately, after slowly weaning off of it for almost a year, last year I had a severe car accident where I had brain trauma causing seizures. They put me back on Clonazepan to control the seizures. I've been on it ever since. Do your homework and find some non-toxic herbs or homeopathic remedies that can help with your symptoms until you can bring your body back into balance with the tools described in this book.

It took years to get cancer. A cancerous malignant tumor is the body's last ditch effort to protect itself. It forms a cocoon around the malignant cells. Is it the wisest thing to do to stick a needle in the protective shell letting the body's last protection be compromised? I'll never forget a conversation with my husband's VA oncologist just before he died in 1994. He said some day needle biopsies will be looked upon as unfavorably as the old practice of "bleeding" very sick patients in a last ditch effort to try to save them. Well, seventeen years have passed and standard medical procedure still includes needle biopsies. You have time to investigate your alternatives. Chemotherapy, radiation and surgery should be a last resort. Save them for last. Don't let fear, your family or your doctor rush you into doing anything that you haven't researched.

Ask questions like, how much chemotherapy can my immune system tolerate? Chemotherapy has devastating toxic side effects. How many months does radiation prolong my life? It's not years. Ask the question! How much does radiation spread the cancer? Is it really worth the risk of spreading the cancer? Is surgery able to get it all? Are you able to "clear the margins"? These are questions that need to be asked. If you can't ask these tough questions bring someone with you that can. Bring someone not afraid to hear the answers, ask the tough questions and take notes. Take a tape recorder or use your iPhone. Get 3 opinions from different orthodox (allopathic) medical doctors and three opinions from holistic, alternative, or homeopathic practitioners that specialize in nontoxic methods of cleansing the years of toxic waste built up in your body to strengthen your immune system to fight the cancer itself.

Many cancers, left totally untreated, have a 5 year "success" rate for 33% of the people. You have time. Most cancer patients die from the side effects of the cut (surgery), burn (radiation), or poison (chemotherapy) methods that your poor doctors are sworn to use by law. Most of the oncologists I've ever met told me they would never subject themselves, friends and particularly family members to these devastating treatments. I used to be Director of Gerontological Services for a hospital. I dealt with oncology and hospice regularly.

Sometimes your own family is very afraid for you. They push you very hard to do traditional treatments hoping you'll be the "one in a million" that gets cured. I've seen just the opposite with my husband after chemotherapy and radiation his scar tissue was too thick with adhesions for the surgeon to operate to buy him that extra month.

Remember cancer and other chronic diseases are big money, big business, a trillion dollar a year industry. Doctors have bills to pay, wives to support, and car payments to make just like us. There's very little money in holistic medicine. Drugs are the biggest money of all. Pharmaceutical representatives make sure medical doctors are kept up to date on the latest drugs.

Do some research on the internet about alternative treatments: IV therapy, whole food vitamin supplements, enzymes, oxygen therapy, diet, exercise, Vitamin C therapy, laetrile, soft laser therapy, homeopathic imprinter therapy, colonics, ionic footbaths, radiation hormesis... the list is endless.

Come to Dr. Lubecki's office to see what worked for me. It's all natural, noninvasive protocols. It might just save your life as it did mine. I was given three months to live and it has now been four years and I'm still going strong.

DISCLAIMER

The author would like it to be clearly understood that she is not involved in any kind of research and does not offer any advice on how sickness should be treated. She is only *reporting* on new discoveries which have been made in holistic medicine and on the way health problems are being successfully prevented in European holistic health clinics.

The opinions expressed in this book are not those of the author. This book is an attempt to synthesize from the available information that which appears to be most relevant and valid.

In this country, all harmless unorthodox treatments are suppressed, leaving only surgery and drugs to choose from. It is the opinion of many leading holistic researchers who use natural therapies, that orthodox treatments often do far more harm than good. They may exhaust the patient's body to such a degree that recovery is no longer possible.

All statements made in this book with regard to the causes of sickness and to the effective nutritional and other natural methods of treatment are well documented as can be seen from the references. The purpose of this book is to provide a synopsis of the available information, thereby cutting this mass of data down to size and making it more easily accessible to the layman.

It has been said that, "A solution to every conceivable problem has already been found by someone, somewhere. The reason we don't know about it is because of lack of communication". This book is an attempt to help patients, as well as those who want to prevent sickness, find the information they are seeking more easily, instead of having to wade through an endless mass of literature on the subject.

Most of the material presented has been taken from the books whose names are listed at the end of this volume.

Unless otherwise indicated, the information in this text is derived from these books. The reader is strongly urged to read them. Lack of space makes it impossible to cover all aspects of sickness as fully as necessary. To make this work concise and easy to read, the author has attempted to explain only the most important features of the holistic treatments available. These books provide more detailed information on most of the topics mentioned.

The majority of the books named can be found on the internet and in your local library or health food store.

CHAPTER 1

⌘

THE THREE BUR HOLES
IN MY SKULL!

I would first like to briefly relate how I miraculously recovered from life threatening health problems thanks to the new discoveries explained in this book. These discoveries quite literally saved my life, when modern medicine no longer gave me any hope.

My first experience with major, life threatening health issues came in 1997. That winter I was plagued with a severe cough and when this would not go away the doctor finally ordered an MRI of my chest. He thought there might be fluid in my lungs.

The MRI showed a moderate sized malignant tumor in the upper lobe of my left lung. The cancer seemed to be well contained and the doctor told me that the best thing to do was to have it surgically removed. To get to the tumor the surgeon had to remove two ribs but the surgery was a success and I soon recovered. Within a month I was back to work and feeling reasonably well so I opted out of chemotherapy.

After that the doctor was concerned that the cancer could return so he asked me to come back once a year for a chest x-ray and a thorough checkup.

Everything went well until the year 2007. When I went in for my usual examination in January of that year I told the doctor that I was experiencing slight shooting pains in the left side of my head, just above and slightly behind my left eye. The doctor said that it was probably nothing, but he would also order an MRI of my head together with the usual x-ray of my chest.

Two days later the doctor called me and said he was

very concerned. They had found three tumors in my brain in the area of the pain. Two were the size of a fried egg and the third one was attached to the bone which forms the forehead. The doctor said that they had probably been growing slowly for some time.

I was told that it was important to find out whether the tumors were malignant so a biopsy was scheduled for the end of the week. Since the only way to access the tumors and obtain a specimen was through my skull the specialist said that they would have to make a tiny bur hole in my skull. They could then put a needle through this hole and obtain the specimen they needed.

I was given a list of the risks of a brain tumor biopsy. They include, but are not limited to: bleeding, infection, CSF (cerebral spinal fluid) leak, stroke, coma, paralysis, weakness, loss of vision, bowel or bladder dysfunction, neurologic deterioration and even death.

Understanding these risks I signed the surgical consent form. My hand shook so badly I had difficulty holding the pen. But there was nothing to be done, there was no alternative.

When I woke up after the biopsy they said that there had been complications. Instead of making only one bur hole they had had to make three bur holes in my skull. This was chiefly due to the large size of the tumors and also to the fact that some of the biopsy specimens they had taken were non-diagnostic.

The final pathological diagnosis: Ana plastic Oligodendroglioma (WHO Grade III).

From then on there was nothing but trouble. I began having terrible headaches and fluid began building up around the tumors. I was so dizzy, walls kept banging into me.

The doctors said that to control the inflammation I would have to be given steroids every day. That was the only way that the swelling could be reduced to prevent brain damage which could cause me to lose consciousness and possibly even die. This continued for the next seven months. Nobody should be given steroids for that long. The side effects were horrific.

They told me that I had three options: radiation, chemotherapy or surgery. Surgery was too risky because of the size of the tumors, which also had tentacles penetrating surrounding areas. Surgery was the only way that the swelling could be reduced, but that could leave me severely disabled and there was no guarantee that the tumors could be entirely removed. I could also become blind, paralyzed and unable to speak. There was no guarantee that this would prolong my life either.

My best option was radiation. Combined with heavy doses of chemotherapy, radiation was most likely to kill the tumors. But there was a danger that it could also cause serious damage to my brain. The radiologist told me that whole brain radiation would also only extend my life by a few months.

After extensive consideration of the possible side effects I began investigating alternative treatments. I started my investigation on the internet. As I discovered alternative therapies and clinics I began calling them for more information. Most of the clinics were very informative but refused to treat me because brain tumors have three problems: the blood brain barrier, confines of the skull and the rapid rate of progression. Many of the treatments would not pass through the blood brain barrier, others exploded the tumors and could not be done within the confines of the skull, while others were too slow, taking months to show results.

My first stop on my journey to wellness was Issels Medical Center in Santa Barbara. I stayed there for one month and learned about healthy organic eating and how the different systems of the body function properly if the energy pathways are clear of harmful toxins and waste matter. I learned more there in one month than I had learned in a lifetime. Why can't our schools teach these things to our children so they could make educated choices about their health?

Particularly, what goes in our mouths and on our skin is so important. We had a lecture for one hour and a half every day as we received Vitamin C, Hydrogen Peroxide and Hydrochloric Acid IV drips. We also had full body massages, lymphatic massages, acupuncture, hyperbaric chamber treatments, far infrared saunas and cooking classes. All this as well as eating a wonderful, nutritious lunch and drinking fresh juices daily.

I wanted to stay there forever; but, to everyone's great disappointment, my tumors remained the same size. I knew that it was the right decision for me to stay there at the time; but, I also knew that I needed to continue my search for a cure.

I had spiritual and motivational counseling at Issels that was phenomenal and I stayed in a wonderful condominium with other patients. We formed lifetime friendships as we walked on the beach together. If you ever have an extra $30,000 I highly recommend Issels to rebuild, rejuvenate and learn about proper health. You have to rebuild your immune system and learn how to cook good tasting healthy foods. Dr. Issels, Dr, Kim, Dr. Danielson, Dr. Lewis, Suzanne Landry (nutritionist) and the entire staff are fabulous. They gave me my first feeling of joy, hope and laughter since my diagnosis. God bless them all.

From the Issels Clinic I went to Mexico where I visited five clinics, none of which gave me much hope. At best a 50% chance of recovery at Hoxsey Clinic. So once again I began their protocol. The black tonic that I drank every day made me so sick that I quickly abandoned it. I was supposed to take it for five years. The cost of the other treatment facilities would also be prohibitive and everything had to be paid for in advance.

Since Mexico was so far and would cost so much I decided to go home. I wanted to die with my family. I began going to a local holistic clinic for vitamin therapy, massages and other natural therapies. I also began to follow a diet of mostly organic raw foods and juices.

Another MRI was scheduled for the beginning of July. It showed that the growth of the tumors had been arrested, but they had not reduced either and were still the same size. The doctor said that at any moment the pressure of the tumors could cause me to pass out. Once that happened I would probably never wake up again.

The doctor kept urging me to have radiation at once. He said that radiation and chemotherapy were my last chance. Previously, when I told him I wanted to go to Mexico he exclaimed that I would "probably come back in a body bag".

What I needed were hope and inspiration, instead, all I saw in the oncology department were the faces of fear, and the smell of death was everywhere.

That biopsy was the biggest mistake I ever made. It was a lot worse than the cancer and it caused so much damage I nearly died. It left me so weak that if I had agreed to the radiation and chemo I would most certainly not be alive today. Also, as a result of the swelling caused by the biopsy, which was done to supposedly save my life, I was given the steroids which ruined my bones and my teeth and damaged my health terribly.

I wish I had known of the alternative treatments sooner. If I had started on them before the biopsy I feel certain I would never have had any problems and by now I would have forgotten that I ever had cancer.

CHAPTER 2
⌘
A RAY OF HOPE

It was a hot summer day in early August. I was lying in bed with the most awful headache imaginable and feeling so weak and depressed that I did not have the strength to get up. The last words of the cancer specialist in the hospital kept ringing in my ears, "if you don't have radiation at once, the pressure of the tumors on your brain has to cause you to pass out and you may never wake up again". Clearly, unless a miracle happened, there was no hope left. Fear set in like an unwelcome houseguest.

Suddenly, the phone rang and brought me out of my daze. It was Val my friend from San Francisco. She wanted to come and visit me and also show me a new book on cancer she had found. Its author was a Dolores Geisler. In this book, entitled "Let's Put an End to Cancer", Dolores explains how she recovered from terminal cancer when she began using new alternative methods.

Dolores had cancer four times: cancer of the uterus, cancer of the ovaries, breast cancer and finally bone cancer. When it came back for the fourth time, she was told that her case was hopeless and there was no longer anything that could be done for her. She had a total of thirty seven surgeries, including two complete, radical mastectomies.

As a result of the steroids and drugs she had been given Dolores gained an enormous amount of weight. She now tipped the scales at over two hundred and fifty pounds. Before the cancers her normal weight was only one hundred and thirty.

When she began using the new alternative methods Dolores recovered rapidly and over the next two years her weight returned back to her usual one hundred and thirty pounds.

Five years have now passed and Dolores has had no further cancer. She writes, "I am beginning to believe that these discoveries make sickness impossible. Try them and see what you think."

In her book Dolores explains that already many years ago scientists in Great Britain discovered that thousands of cells become malignant in our bodies all the time. This means that we all have cancer from the day we are born, we just know nothing about it because the malignant cells are immediately destroyed and taken care of by our immune system.

As a result it is now known that it is unlikely to have cancer or tumors if a person's body is regularly cleansed of toxins and their immune system is strong. These doctors believe that tumors can only develop if a person's body becomes excessively toxic and their immune system is so weak that it can no longer cope with the constant influx of new cancerous cells.

Cancer is a symptom that the body has become overloaded with different toxins and the immune system is failing and can no longer destroy the thousands of new malignant cells fast enough. So called malignant tumors are not some kind of disease which can only be treated by specialists with cut and burn methods, the way that we are led to believe.

The purpose of the new alternative methods for treating malignancies is, therefore, not so much to destroy tumors or treat the malignancy itself in any way, but to strengthen and cleanse the body to help it fight the cancer. It has been found that if this can be done, before it is too late and too much damage has occurred, the body has no trouble in dealing with the malignancy. Often even large tumors disappear within a short time.

ONLY THE BODY ITSELF HAS THE ABILITY TO DESTROY MALIGNANT CELLS, <u>WITHOUT HARMING HEALTHY CELLS.</u>

All manmade attempts at trying to destroy tumors and cancer cells inevitably weaken the immune system terribly and damage healthy tissues. As a result, they often do far more harm than the cancer. That explains why although billions of dollars have been spent on cancer research and the government has given enormous grants for this purpose, absolutely no progress whatsoever has been made and no solution to cancer has been found for close to a hundred years.

We are now no closer to finding a cure for malignancies than we were when cancer research first started. More people are dying of this horrible disease all the time and the so called cures that have been tried have been a total disaster. These cures do more harm and kill more people than they supposedly save. Early detection techniques make it appear as though people are living longer.

This is because there is nothing anyone can do to stop the body from continually producing more malignant cells and it is also impossible to find a safe way of destroying malignant cells without destroying or damaging healthy cells. Only our own immune system has no trouble in doing this.

ONLY THE BODY ITSELF IS EQUIPPED TO DEAL WITH THE MALIGNANT CELLS. NO MANMADE CURE FOR CANCER HAS EVER BEEN FOUND TO BE TRULY SUCCESSFUL.

The chief purpose of the new alternative/holistic methods are not so much to destroy the tumors but to cleanse the body, strengthen the immune system and remove anything that is known to weaken the body's natural defenses. Common sense tells us that if this can be done it is impossible to have malignancies and cancers which are not too advanced can be easily controlled and eradicated from the body.

Already before the Second World War Dr. Max Gerson, the famous pioneer in natural treatments for cancer, said, when testifying before a Senate Subcommittee in Washington, D.C.: "Early cancers and skin cancers are easy to treat". Dr. Gerson used fresh juices, coffee enemas and other natural means to cleanse the body and strengthen the immune system. His success made him very unpopular with the medical profession so his license to practice was revoked and he had to escape to Mexico and open a clinic there. Later his nurse poisoned him with arsenic but not before he published his famous book <u>A Cancer Therapy, Results of Fifty Cases.</u>

When I read Dolores' book I felt a new surge of hope. Perhaps everything was not lost yet and there was still a faint chance that I might get well again. But where was I to find a holistic clinic or doctor who would have the equipment Dolores writes about and who also knew what to do?

SUMMARY

Clearly, a cure for cancer has never been found. All those poor experimental animals which have been tortured to death in the most awful manner died in vain. The same is true of the billions which have been spent on cancer research. All that money has simply been dumped into greedy pockets. The only thing that has been achieved by all this is that chemotherapy, radiation and surgery have tortured to death more people than our country ever lost in all the wars it was ever engaged in.

Malignancies can be treated successfully with the natural procedures explained in the following chapters. The best proof is that if these alternative methods are used properly the body itself, without any help from anyone else, sometimes breaks down malignant tumors so fast that a big improvement can be seen from one day to the next.

CHAPTER 3
⌘
Dr. Lubecki – Initial Visit

After reading Dolores' book, together with Val we began calling everyone and anyone who we thought might know of the methods mentioned by her. We called holistic clinics, doctors, health food stores, but without any success. Nobody seemed to know what we were talking about.

Finally, after numerous attempts and failures, we managed to locate a small clinic which appeared to have what we were looking for. I made an appointment for the next day.

When the girl at the front desk heard that I had cancer she looked very alarmed and told me that their office did not treat cancer patients. She suggested that I call the hospital and see a cancer specialist there.

"But I do not want to be treated for cancer", I answered in despair. "I only want to cleanse my body of heavy metals, toxins and parasites".

That seemed to calm her down a little and when I had filled out the usual forms she called the doctor.

After he had listened to my story the doctor said: "We do not treat malignancies in this clinic. We are not allowed to do so. I would find myself behind bars if there was the slightest suspicion that I had treated someone for cancer, or that I had said that I could cure or help their cancer."

"If I tell anyone that I can help them or that I could cure their problem by using natural methods I am breaking the law and I could lose my license or go to jail. They could accuse me of misleading people, causing fatal delays or even causing someone's death. However," the doctor continued, "you will be glad to know that we do use the kind of methods you are looking for."

The doctor then went on to explain that, "in Europe they have found that if the body can be cleansed of mercury, nickel, cadmium and other chemicals by using the homeopathic imprinter and a large, low level laser the immune system begins to function better again. If the treatment is started in time, the cancer disappears automatically without any treatments directly for the cancer or the tumors."

"This is because they have found that cadmium, nickel, mercury and other chemicals weaken the immune system more than anything. As a result, they make it impossible for it to defend the body from cancer."

"Once these poisons no longer interfere with normal function the immune system becomes strong again and it has no problem in dealing with the cancer, the way it has been designed to do since the beginning of time."

"Don't ever tell anyone that I said so, but getting rid of your brain tumors should be a piece of cake", he added. "Hopefully, if you can keep your body free of metals, chemicals and other toxins the cancer will never come back. This is especially true if you can also do all you can to keep your immune system healthy and strong. These new discoveries now make it a lot easier to help the body get rid of the cancer and other chronic health problems."

"Cancer of the brain seems to be the easiest of all cancers for the body to get rid of. This is probably because the brain has the richest blood supply".

"But, before we do anything, you have to sign a form which states that you clearly understand that any treatments you may receive in this clinic are not for cancer in any way. The only purpose of our treatments is to improve your overall health. These treatments are not for any specific condition, especially not for cancer."

I was stunned by what he had said; nobody had ever

said anything like this before. I kept being told that my case was hopeless and that I could die any moment. Even the Mexican cancer clinics only gave me a fifty percent chance of survival, at best and most of them said no to brain tumors because they grow too fast.

CHAPTER 4

⌘

FIRST STEP DETOX

The doctor explained that the first thing we had to do was to remove bacteria, viruses, parasites and chemicals from my body. He said that it has been found in Europe that this can now be done in just a few seconds by using a homeopathic imprinter in a new way (this is described in more detail in Chapter 7).

The doctor first placed my hand on the INPUT plate of the homeopathic imprinter and imprinted the greatly magnified vibrations in my hand on a small, black, plastic box that contained the homeopathic remedy, which he had placed on the OUTPUT plate of the imprinter.

It is important to understand that the electro-magnetic vibrations of everything that may be in our body spread throughout the body like an electric current. As a result, the hand contains the vibrations of everything in the entire body. Therefore, when the vibrations in the hand are imprinted on the homeopathic remedy, which is in the plastic box, then the remedy contains the greatly magnified vibrations of everything that may be in the body at that time: chemicals, viruses, parasites, and bacteria.

The doctor then reversed this order and placed the remedy on the INPUT plate and my hand on the OUTPUT plate. He said that by doing this it is now possible to send our own tremendously magnified vibrations back through our body. When these magnified vibrations pass through our tissues they immediately kill all viruses, bacteria and parasites as well as neutralizing or removing many chemicals.

After this the doctor placed me under a large low level (soft) laser which he said he had purchased in Switzerland. In that country they had told him that such a laser removes or neutralizes heavy metals---especially important in the case of cancer patients being mercury, nickel and cadmium. These three have been found to be just about the most carcinogenic (cancer causing) substances on earth. They are now frequently found in jewelry, watches, rings, dental restorations (crowns, fillings, partials) and even in such processed foods as: gums, chocolates, toothpastes, cosmetic. Because our planet is so terribly polluted it is not unusual to find that even vegetables and health foods can be polluted with cancer causing chemicals.

When we had finished using the imprinter and the laser an assistant took me to another room where I spent over half an hour with my feet in an ionic foot bath. The purpose was to detoxify my body as fast as possible. She also placed the pads of two Metatron Electric Stimulators (see later chapter) on different parts of my body. She said that this would speed up healing and enhance the cleansing effect of the ionic foot bath also decreasing many of the side effects of rapid detoxification (headache, nausea, and fatigue).

The doctor explained that the most important thing was to remove all the different factors which were interfering with the energy flow in my body. Therefore, as explained in more detail in later chapters, I also had my atlas vertebra adjusted, I was taught how to eliminate my allergies and the effects of harmful past events and, finally, how to treat my scars.

There was an almost immediate improvement. When I woke up the next day to my surprise and relief my arms and legs were no longer numb and painful and my headache was better. Within a few weeks, I could also drive again, something I had not been able to do for the last seven months.

To help cleanse my body faster I went back to the clinic three or four times a week for the ionic foot baths. Each time they put the pads of two Metatron Electrical Stimulators on different parts of my body. The latter device has two large pads which are placed on the skin. Using this form of electrical stimulation has been found to enormously speedup healing and cleansing. It helps clear the excess toxins out of the blood and lymphatic systems.

There was a steady improvement. I again began going for long walks, my headaches were a lot better and I felt stronger every day. I was no longer paralyzed on my right side as I had been many times before.

I went in for my MRI at the end of October full of hope. I truly expected they would tell me my tumors were either gone or at least a lot better.

Following the visit to the alternative doctor I bought my own homeopathic imprinter together with the hand held laser and the enhancer. Now that I finally had this important equipment, I began treating myself several times a day.

SUMMARY

As already explained, European doctors have found that cancer can only develop if the immune system is compromised because the body is contaminated with metals and chemicals---the most carcinogenic of these being cadmium, nickel and mercury. When these are removed or neutralized with the low level laser and other chemicals are removed or neutralized by using the homeopathic imprinter, the immune system becomes stronger and it can again begin fighting off the cancer.

This is, obviously, only true as long as the cancer is not too advanced and the body has not been too badly damaged by the treatments used by modern medicine.

In Europe it is believed that if the laser and the imprinter become widely used to prevent contamination with chemicals, cancer would cease to exist. This is also true of many of the other health problems which are caused by chemicals and infections: MS, Alzheimer's, rheumatoid arthritis, many allergies, amputations due to infections, many skin problems and other degenerative, metabolic and autoimmune diseases.

CHAPTER 5
✤
DISASTER!
MY MRI NO BETTER

Following the MRI they told me to come back to the clinic in three days. They would then tell me the results and whether there was any change or not.

I was so impatient and anxious to know what they had found on the MRI that I called the clinic the next day to ask if perhaps they already knew the results. They answered that there had been a delay and asked me to call again the following day. To my surprise this time they just briefly told me that there was no change. "The tumors were there just like before".

It is hard to describe my disappointment. I felt as if the ground had fallen out from under my feet and for the rest of that day I walked around in a dismal mood. All my hopes had been shattered.

When I woke up the next morning I felt better for the night's rest and I began thinking that there had to be a mistake. I felt so much better, I was able to go for long walks, and my pain was gone. It seemed impossible that the tumors were no better.

When I went to the clinic the following day they dismissed me quickly by briefly telling me that my condition was stable and that I should come back for another evaluation in three months.

They did not measure the tumors, the way they had always done in the past, and they did not tell me that I could die at any moment, the way they had also always done every time they had seen me before. They just said, "Come back in three months for another evaluation." I was then given copies of the last two MRI's and they sent me home.

As soon as I arrived I ran to the computer and I began looking at the two MRI's. Brain tumors appear like a whitish cloud on the MRI. The tumors could be clearly seen on the first MRI. They were huge, as big as fried eggs.

On the second MRI there was no white cloud. Was I making a mistake or was the tumor gone?

I then took the MRI to some of the alternative clinics I had previously visited. Opinions varied. Some of them said that they were afraid to give a definite opinion but others said that it was not impossible that all that was left was some diffuse scarring which made it look as if the tumor was still there, especially when a contrast medium was used. Another opinion was that what was left of the tumors were the capsules which the body had formed around the malignant cells.

I waited for another two and a half months before having any more tests to monitor my progress. This time I went to Toronto, Canada, to the ONCO labs and had what is called the AMAS test which is believed to be the most accurate test for cancer. To my great relief the test came back negative and I was told that I had no active cancer any more.

The next MRI was scheduled for early February. I had to wait almost two weeks for the results because my doctor's mother was dying so the doctor was too busy to look at my MRI.

Finally, there was a message on my phone from the hospital which stated, "Congratulations! Your tumor has changed". The MRI showed that the tumor, or what was left of it, was no longer picking up the contrast. A great deal of healing and improvement had taken place since the last MRI three months previously.

PREVENTION IS THE ONLY WAY TO GO

Dealing with cancer and then trying to recover from the treatments is like playing with fire. Don't wait until you already have cancer, do everything that is in this book to prevent cancer.

Even if I have no more problems with the tumors, I still have to get over the effects of the steroids which have left me with severe osteoporosis. Then there are also the effects of the biopsies which left damage due to the scaring and hemorrhaging they caused.

The devastating effects of the steroids did not show up until several months after I was finally off them. My doctor warned me that if I discontinued the steroids too rapidly this could cause my blood pressure to drop so low that I could die. As a result, I was on heavy doses of steroids not only for the seven months that I had the brain cancer, but it took another five months to gradually get off them.

About two months after I was finally able to discontinue the steroids the pain started. I was in agony for months. The steroids had not only destroyed my bones and my teeth but they had also caused serious damage to my joints and other tissues. The pain was so bad that at times it was difficult to walk and sleeping was impossible. It took several months of daily soft laser treatments before there was enough improvement for the pain to become manageable. If it had not been for the soft or low level laser, I truly believe that the bone loss and pain could have crippled or even killed me.

Then came the seizures. In early July for some unknown reason I suddenly had a seizure soon after waking up from a nap in the afternoon. Next day the seizures became a lot worse and more frequent. They were thought to be due to the tumor so another MRI was immediately scheduled.

I was put on anti-seizure drugs but these caused such a violent reaction that I had to discontinue them. I vomited endlessly and my entire body turned red. The following day I had over a hundred seizures almost one after another. I felt certain I was going to end up in the hospital or dead.

I went back to my holistic doctor who said I should try lying on a strong magnetic pad and use a new low-level laser. The following day I only had three seizures. Within the next two days the seizures stopped altogether and I was able to return to the land of the living again. It was like a miracle. I had managed to cheat death once again.

The only problems, due to the medical treatments, that I still had not recovered from were weakness, ringing in the ears all day and night and continual weight loss. My weight dropped to one hundred and five pounds and I began fearing the worst again. It was a great relief, therefore, when a few months later I gradually gained fifteen pounds and my weight returned back to normal.

I wish I had known what I now know before all this started. With the new methods, described in this book, all my problems could have been easily prevented.

CHAPTER 6

⌘

THE SOFT LASERS

The discovery of the wonderful healing properties of laser therapy has simplified health care enormously. Laser therapy may not only speed up recovery tremendously but sometimes it may even make it possible to help patients with conditions for which there appeared to be no cure in the past. The short case histories at the end of the first half of this chapter will give a better idea of the amazing healing power of lasers.

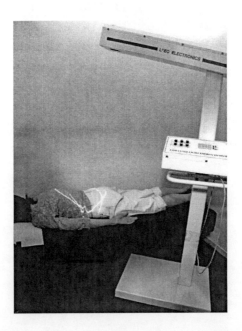

The large soft or low level laser, which the alternative doctor placed me under, is widely used in Europe and doctors have found that when a higher setting is used heavy metals are neutralized or removed from the body. It is well known that once the heavy metals, especially nickel, mercury and cadmium, have been removed or neutralized by using the laser many cancers stop growing and soon begin to disappear.

The doctors found that if the laser is used together with the homeopathic imprinter virtually all early cancers and even some more advanced cancers rapidly reverse and tumors may soon begin to go away. In some cases the tumors shrink so fast that a big improvement can be seen from one day to the next.

This is the main reason why it is believed in Europe that cancer is primarily caused by the body's sensitivity or allergy to the heavy metals mercury, nickel and cadmium. These doctors have found that it is much more difficult to develop tumors or cancer if the large laser and the imprinter are used regularly for prevention.

From this we can see that nobody has to have cancer any more. We could put an end to cancer at once, if we really wanted to do so. Unfortunately, too many individuals and organizations are heavily committed to keeping things the way they are. Consequently, they will do everything they can to resist change.

Case history #1   Our son was born with a large cyst in his brain. He made no response when spoken to and just stared vacantly into space. We were told that the only solution was surgery, but they warned us that surgery could result in serious brain damage. On the suggestion of a friend we tried laser treatments twice a day. Within two months all signs of the cyst disappeared and an MRI showed that it had shrunk to half its size. Our son now appears to be quite normal.

Case history #2   I had a severe case of psoriasis and my entire body was covered in large lesions. The treatments that we tried helped very little or not at all. After a month of laser treatments twice a day the psoriasis disappeared and has not come back

Case history #3   In the summer of 1998 I woke up one morning to find that I could hardly raise my left arm. By next day it was completely paralyzed. I consulted many doctors, none of whom could find the cause of the problem. MRIs, CT scans and numerous other tests showed nothing. When there was no improvement for three months, on the advice of a friend, I went to have a laser treatment, without really believing it could possibly do any good. But it only took ten minutes and cost a mere forty dollars, so why not? To my utter amazement when I woke up the next morning I noticed some movement in my arm and within a month I was back to normal. There is now no difference in the strength of my two arms. Ten years have passed and there hasn't been any recurrence of the problem.

HAND HELD LASERS

The large laser described above has its own stand, which measures about six feet in height. This laser can be set higher for removing or neutralizing heavy metals, or lower for healing and relief of pain. The hand held lasers function at only one level and they cannot be used for removing heavy metals unless an enhancer is used. However, hand held lasers still have a wonderful healing and stimulating effect.

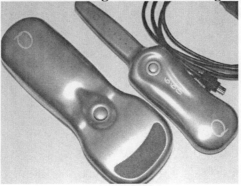

The User's Manual for these lasers shows many specific applications which have been tried successfully for various conditions. However, by far the best results can be obtained if the entire body is scanned regularly. This should be done twice a day, or even more than that in emergencies. For instance, if a person is in pain the laser may reduce or even stop the pain if it is used enough. Special attention should be given to scars, stretch marks, tattoos and calluses. The laser should be used for a few seconds longer over these areas.

Regular treatments with the hand held laser can result in: an amazing increase in the strength of muscles, an improvement in the function of the organs, steady weight loss, disappearance of calluses, and regeneration of nerves, muscles, ligaments, bone and soft tissues. Other benefits may be an improvement in the appearance of wrinkles and scars, better eyesight, better hearing and a lot more.

After you have used the laser for a time you will realize that it is possible to enjoy good health if you scan your entire body twice a day with a laser. I use the laser for nine minutes every morning and evening and sometimes also at different times during the day.

EASTERN MEDICINE AND THE LASER

Thousands of years ago doctors of Eastern Medicine discovered that as long as nothing is interfering with the energy flow in the body it is impossible to have many health problems. In China and other Eastern countries people went to their doctor not when they were already sick, the way we are accustomed to doing, but to prevent health problems.

The doctor's job was to remove interference with the energy flow in the patient's body before symptoms appeared. Therefore, the doctor was only paid as long as his patients remained well. If a patient became ill the doctor would have to treat him for nothing, because it was considered the doctor's fault that his patient was sick. He had failed to remove interference with the energy flow in his patient's body in time. The doctor had to treat the patient for nothing until he had recovered.

Acupuncture is used to boost the energy flow in a patient's body and speed up his recovery, ease his pain and a host of other benefits. Doctors who use lasers have found that scanning the body with the small hand held laser has a similar, or perhaps sometimes an even stronger effect than having acupuncture treatments. When the laser is used the flow of energy in the body improves tremendously and the entire body becomes stronger and begins to function better.

If the laser is used regularly together with the homeopathic imprinter and the other methods explained in this book, it is much less likely you will have health problems. Providing of course that you also get adjusted (see CH 12), eat sensibly, exercise regularly, take the necessary supplements and look after your health as best you can. It is best to start doing all this while you are well and not wait until damage has been done.

SUMMARY

If you are truly concerned about staying well you have to try to find a doctor who has a large laser. This may present a serious problem. There are very few doctors in the USA who have such lasers or have any experience in using them.

In this country we are used to going to a doctor only when we are already sick, or in so much pain that we can't stand it any longer. Consequently, by the time we finally begin looking for help, so many things may have gone wrong and so much damage may have been done that it could be difficult for even the best doctor to get us well quickly, or even get us well at all.

If we are to stay well everyone has to take charge and responsibility for his own health and try to learn how to correct as many problems as possible by himself. If you can do the things explained in this book you will avoid many health complications.

Finally, if you are truly interested in your health and you want to do everything possible to stay well you have to purchase a small hand held laser and scan your entire body twice a day. If you do not do this it is more difficult to keep the body balanced and functioning normally. If you also use the enhancer, this will have the same effect as using the large laser in a doctor's office. When the hand held laser is used together with the enhancer it also neutralizes or removes the heavy metals, in a way similar to the large laser described above. The difference is that the large laser only takes two or three minutes to do the job, while the hand held laser takes longer.

When using the small, hand held laser and the enhancer to remove heavy metals you should scan your head, the neck and the upper body, down to just above the nipple line, for four or five minutes or more, every day. You should hold the enhancer (660) about six inches from the skin and move it slowly in small clockwise circles. Spend more time over the teeth which have fillings, crowns or other metal restorations.

NOTE - You should not miss reading the chapter on lasers in Dolores Geisler's book. She writes about many people who recovered from apparently hopeless, incurable conditions when the laser was used. There are some excellent photos.

CHAPTER 7
⌘
THE HOMEOPATHIC IMPRINTER

LEARNING HOW TO USE THE HOMEOPATHIC IMPRINTER CORRECTLY IS THE SINGLE MOST IMPORTANT THING THAT YOU HAVE TO DO IF YOU WANT TO STAY WELL AND PREVENT HEALTH PROBLEMS

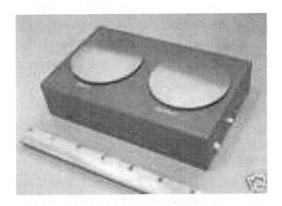

Holistic doctors believe that the new way of using the homeopathic imprinter is by far one of the most important discoveries ever made in healing. The new method enables us to do many things which it was difficult, or even impossible, to do in the past.

For instance, so far we have not been able to find a cure for viruses. There is no drug and even the body itself has problems in dealing with viruses. Viral conditions, the best known are probably CFS (chronic fatigue syndrome) and herpes, often lingered endlessly, sometimes for years.

Amazingly, European doctors have found that when the homeopathic imprinter is used the new way it kills all viruses INSTANTLY! Therefore, if the homeopathic imprinter is correctly used viral infections cannot occur. This alone would eliminate many conditions.

The discovery of antibiotics a hundred years ago was hailed as a great breakthrough. But antibiotics seem to be becoming less and less effective. It is believed that bacteria are developing resistance to antibiotics and they are no longer killed by these drugs. In some cases it has even been found that taking the drug can actually make an infection worse. It is believed that the most likely reason for this is that antibiotics also kill the friendly bacteria in our gut and this weakens our immune system even more. Another problem is that antibiotics can sometimes also produce nasty side effects. There have even been some rare cases where people have even died or developed serious health problems after using antibiotics.

This cannot happen with the new method of using the imprinter. If properly used the imprinter kills all bad bacteria instantly. There is no bacterial infection it does not get rid of at once, quite regardless of how bad the infection may be. There are never any side effects of any kind.

If the homeopathic imprinter ever becomes widely used this would save countless millions of lives and billions in expenses. For instance, far more Americans have died from hospital acquired infections than from all the wars this country has ever taken part in. Hospital acquired infections are the fourth leading cause of death and doctors can often do nothing to help. None of these people would have to die if the imprinter was used.

Many amputations, usually the legs, are also the result of the inability of antibiotics to control infections. Nobody would have to have their legs amputated from infections if the imprinter became widely used.

European doctors have also found that when used the new way the homeopathic imprinter kills intestinal parasites and some forms of Candida. It also removes or neutralizes many of the chemicals in the body which come from foods, water, deodorants, cosmetics, pesticides and other sources. There are absolutely no side effects as is so often the case with drugs.

If properly used, the imprinter eliminates all infectious conditions caused by bacteria, viruses and parasites. Such conditions may include not only the usual common symptoms we are familiar with, but also often such things as: allergic symptoms, asthma, rheumatoid arthritis and many other problems which it has only recently been discovered can also be caused by micro-organisms.

Since it also removes or neutralizes many chemicals the imprinter can be very helpful in the prevention and treatment of those conditions which are now known to be almost entirely caused by the chemicals which are present in such enormous quantities in our environment and foods. The best examples of these conditions are probably: cancer, Multiple Sclerosis (MS), Alzheimer's, Fibromyalgia, Chronic Fatigue Syndrome (CFS.) and many others.

As already mentioned in the chapter on lasers, European doctors who use this method believe you are a lot less likely to develop cancer, MS, Alzheimer's or any of the other chronic conditions caused by modern chemicals if the imprinter and the laser are used correctly for prevention.

INTESTINAL PARASITES

The ineffectiveness of modern methods for detecting intestinal parasites--worms, Candida, Giardia--is one of the most important reasons for our failure to cope with cancer.

Unfortunately, the commonly used medical procedures for discovering the presence of intestinal parasites are so inaccurate they often do more to deceive the doctor than to help him. As a result, the medical profession has been misled into believing that parasitic infestations are rare and play an insignificant part in causing sickness.

It is only since electro-diagnosis and muscle-testing have begun to be used that the enormities of the problem posed by intestinal parasites have been clearly understood. Electro-diagnosis and muscle-testing are not only more accurate than standard medical tests, they are easier to use. It is no longer necessary to spend several days waiting for the results of lab tests. With electro-diagnosis and muscle-testing it is possible to tell in a matter of seconds whether a person has parasites or not. Since these new methods of diagnosis have begun to be used, it has been found that close to ninety percent of persons tested show signs of parasitic infestation. In the case of cancer patients the figure is even higher. Cancer patients practically always show signs of heavy parasitic infestation, as well as the open ileo-cecal valve syndrome. This is not surprising when one considers that cancer is only a symptom of extreme toxicity. Intestinal parasites and an open ileo-cecal valve cause the body to be subjected to a continuous flood of poisons. In no other way can such quantities of toxins enter the human organism.

The ileo-cecal valve syndrome is probably the most important problem which can be caused by parasites. The ileo-cecal valve (see illustration) is located at the end of the small intestine. Its function is to prevent back flow of the highly toxic fecal matter from the colon. If this happens, a veritable river of poison pours into the body.

Until a few years ago, no one suspected that the ileo-cecal valve could malfunction and become unable to close fully in many people. The only evidence we had that the ileo-cecal valve does not function normally in some people was the evidence gathered from barium studies performed in the case of patients, it could sometimes be seen that the barium had not been stopped by the valve and had penetrated deep into the small intestine. However, the number of patients examined this way was very small. There was no easy, quick way of checking large numbers of people. Therefore, there was no reason to suspect that a malfunctioning ileo-cecal valve could be a common problem. Since muscle-testing has been used, it has been possible to show that in close to half the patients tested the valve does not function normally and remains open all the time. This can be a very serious problem and it can often be one of the main causes of many conditions--such as back pain, headaches, skin conditions or fatigue. In the case of cancer patients a much higher proportion are found to have an open ileo-cecal valve. Not surprisingly, persons who have been diagnosed as having cancer show evidence of an open ileo-cecal valve practically every time.

THE ALIMENTARY CANAL

This short description of the alimentary canal, or gastrointestinal tract, is included so the reader might have a better understanding of the function and importance of the ileo-cecal valve. After mastication (chewing) food passes down the esophagus (or gullet) into the stomach. Comparatively little digestion takes place in the stomach. The main function of this organ is to act as a storage tank from which food is slowly emptied into the small intestine. It is the in small intestine that most digestion takes place. Here the food is acted upon by the pancreatic enzymes and enzymes secreted by tiny glands in the walls of the small intestine itself. These enzymes break the food down into its basic chemical components, which then diffuse through the walls of the small intestine directly into the blood stream.

The total length of the small intestine is about twenty feet. It is divided into three sections, the last of which is called the ileum. The ileo-cecal valve is located at the end of the ileum, at the point where the small intestine empties into the colon. The first part of the colon is called the cecum, hence the name ileo-cecal valve.

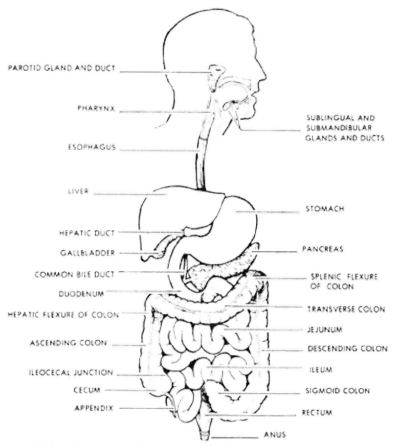

This diagram shows the different component parts of the gastrointestinal tract.

When a certain quantity of fully digested food accumulates in the end of the ileum, the valve relaxes and the end of the food is pushed into the cecum. As soon as the food has passed through, the valve closes firmly behind it. This way the fermenting, putrefying fecal matter in the colon is prevented from backing up into the ileum.

The walls of the colon, or large intestine, are designed in such a remarkable manner that they are impermeable to the poisons inside the colon. Under normal conditions, the only way that these poisons could pass into the blood stream would be if they could somehow get back into the ileum. But this is impossible since the ileo-cecal valve remains closed and does not allow any backup from the colon into the small intestine.

POSSIBLE CAUSES OF AN OPEN ILEO-CECAL VALVE

The reasons why the ileo-cecal valve remains open in some people are not clear and we shall probably never understand exactly what happens. There is no doubt that one of the causes is an energy imbalance. This must be so since the valve can readily be made to function normally again if the energy imbalance is corrected by touching or rubbing the acupuncture points shown at the end of this chapter. Exactly how this acupressure treatment corrects the imbalance of energy and causes the ileo-cecal valve to function normally is a mystery, as is the question of how the Chinese discovered what should be done. It can be easily demonstrated that immediately following the acupressure treatment, the valve always closes and begins to function normally again. As is usual with acupuncture techniques the result is always positive. If this were not so, the Chinese doctors could never have guaranteed their patients' health the way they did.

Another possibility is that if a person has parasites they, somehow, cause the ileo-cecal valve to stay open. How worms can cause the valve to remain open is difficult to understand. Nevertheless, is has been found that almost every person who has an open ileo-cecal valve also shows signs of slight irritation, or inflammation, of the entire abdomen. This irritation is thought to be caused by parasites, since it soon disappears when patients take herbs to kill parasites. Also, even if the acupressure treatment for closing the valve is not used, the ileo-cecal valve will always close once the parasites are gone.

HOW COMMON ARE PARASITES?

Most people are not aware of the danger posed to their health by intestinal parasites. Since lab tests are practically always negative, no matter how severely infested a patient may be, medical doctors seldom mention intestinal parasites. We also rarely see anything in the press concerning health problems caused by parasites. However, if you look in the right places you will find plenty of literature showing that a small minority of specialists are very much aware of the prevalence of parasitic infestation. For instance, in a pamphlet put out by a medical manufacturer in Phoenix, Arizona, we read:

Colon therapy has an anthelminitic action--this means that parasites are removed. We find that over 90 percent of the people we examine in our clinics have some form of parasites. The most common of all are tapeworms. Our skilled technicians report seeing green, brown, grey, yellow, and white ones--and various combinations. Patients report seeing pieces of tapeworm in the toilet bowl, varying in length from a few inches to several feet. The longest one reported was 57 feet. Various other parasites are seen including hookworms, pinworms, whipworms, and many other exotic forms. Tapeworms are usually beef, pork, or fish variety. Many vegetarians also have various parasites. Their eggs may be ingested with vegetables or fruit. Threadworms and hookworms may pass through the unbroken skin; they are sometimes picked up when one walks through the grass.

In a full-page advertisement, with a large photo of a small girl handing a pencil to a classmate, for a vermifuge called Combantrin we read in a New Zealand monthly:

The simple act of passing a pencil, sharing a book, touching the same doorknob, or even sharing a house with untreated adults is all that is required for parasites to spread--no matter how clean your child may be no matter how careful you are. The symptoms caused by parasites may include: loss of appetite, anal and vulvae itching and scratching, disturbed sleep, bloating, occasional bed wetting in younger children, swelling of the face and lymph nodes of the neck, a green or yellowish discharge in the urine, loose bowels, etc. These may seem like common occurrence in childhood, but, unfortunately, this is because the parasite problem is a common one.

I once told a patient that I thought her daily migraines were caused by parasites and an open ileo-cecal valve. I asked her whether she found this very surprising and whether she was aware that parasites are very common and often cause headaches, fatigue, and other symptoms. She answered that she was aware of this since recently she had taken her children to a doctor in Germany because they were complaining of indigestion and restlessness. After examining the children, the doctor told her he found they had pinworms and these parasites were causing their symptoms. At the time she could not believe this. She told the doctor it was impossible for her children to have parasites since she insisted on the highest standard of hygiene. Also, she had not seen any signs of worms in the children's clothes or beds. But the doctor insisted and told her that over 90 percent of people in that area had parasites, so she should not feel embarrassed in any way about her children also having them. When I heard this, I no longer felt bad about telling the lady I thought she had worms. This proved to be the correct diagnosis because when she took the herbs her headaches soon improved. Yet this patient had been to a number of doctors and none of them had been able to do anything for her.

In an interview recorded in a health publication, Dr. William Kelley, the famous cancer specialist says:

> I find parasites in 92 percent of people. Everybody, rich or poor, the whole population has parasites. They are not restricted to the lower classes at all. Pets are great carriers of parasites. Also, vegetables may carry parasitic organisms. One day I had a lady who was a little over 5 feet tall and weighed 300 pounds. She was on a 400-500 calorie diet and starving to death. I said, "You've got so many worms, all you assimilate is water." This horrified her. Most people are upset at the thought of having worms. She started a bottle of special supplements I gave her but nothing happened. So she went to her family doctor who took a stool culture but could find nothing.
> The lady decided to finish the bottle of supplements by taking then regularly. One night she was lying in her bed when she felt a tickling in her throat and thought it was mucous. She went to the bathroom and coughed it up, put it on a Kleenex, turned the light on, looked at it

and screamed, scaring her husband to death. They found the head and two more inches of a tapeworm which had come up in the throat. Lots of times, in children particularly, the tapeworm will come through the nose looking for more to eat.

Parasites mimic a lot of diseases. Like heart trouble. I found this once. I had a nurse as a patient who had suffered with all kinds of heart trouble and went to doctors for years. She had these heart spells.

I said, "You should have gone to a vet."

She said, "Why is that?"

"Because we have found what is wrong with you, you have heart worms."

We put her on a nutritional program and she has had no trouble since. Most stomach aches and colitis have a parasitic involvement. Liver damage and liver trouble can be caused by worms. Sometimes a colony of worms will crawl up in the gall bladder and cause trouble. This can be the problem with many overweight people. The worms are well fed, but the body is only getting the water and the calories and a fraction of the nutrients.

Maurice Messegue, the famous French herbalist writes this about garlic:

> Nowadays statistics indicate that those parts of the world where garlic is eaten in quantity have a low incidence of cancer. Wherever I found garlic in use I found health.
>
> From this statement we see that in areas where people eat a lot of garlic, the best herb for killing parasites, few have worms and an open ileo-cecal valve. As a result, the incidence of cancer is also reduced.

DIARRHEA

Diarrhea is the result of an inflamed condition of the colon. In more extreme cases this condition is called colitis. If ulceration is present the name ulcerative colitis is used. Since this condition can usually be easily corrected by de-worming the patient, some experts have suggested that it is always caused by intestinal parasites. Since all patients with colon cancer have been found to be heavily infested with parasites, it has also been suggested that parasites are probably the only cause of colon cancer.

PROSTATE TROUBLE

Apart from causing difficulty in urination in some cases, inflammation of the prostate gland in men can cause lower back pain, shoulder pain, and other symptoms. Prostate trouble responds so well to large doses of garlic and other herbs which kill parasites, that it appears that in the majority of cases inflammation and swelling of the prostate are caused entirely by parasites. As in the case of colitis, all patients with prostate cancer have been found to be heavily infested with intestinal parasites. Therefore, it has been suggested that parasites are probably the only cause of prostate cancer.

HOW TO CORRECT THE OPEN ILEO-CECAL

This can be done in a matter of seconds by:

1. Rubbing the first point on the spleen meridian (Spleen 1). This point is located on the inside of the large toe, next to the toe nail. (See drawing below.) This must be done on both feet.

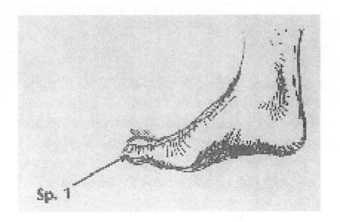

2. Rubbing the third point on the large intestine median. This point is located just below the knuckle of the index finger. This must be done on both hands.

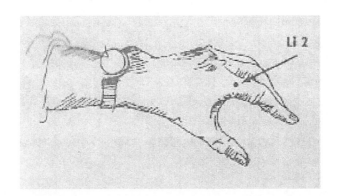

3. Touching (not rubbing) the 58th point on the bladder meridians on both legs at the same time. The point bladder 58 is located on the side of the leg, about two thirds of the way down from the knee to the ankle. (See drawing below.) You must hold your hands straight down the sides of your calves. Fingers together and not separated. The tips of your fingers should be about two inches above your ankles.

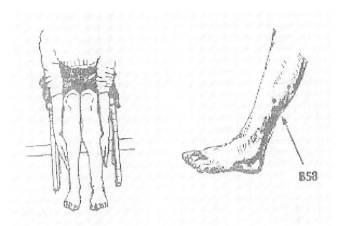

4. Touching (not rubbing) the point bladder 58 on the LEFT leg and at the same time touching (not rubbing) the point Kidney 7 on the RIGHT leg. The point Kidney 7 is located behind and below the ankle.

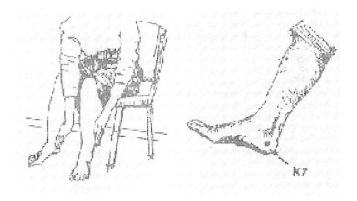

The procedure can be carried out either by the patient himself or by another person. As is usual with acupuncture, the result is always the same. Every time the above mentioned points are treated, the open ileo-cecal valve corrects itself instantly. This shows that if acupuncture points are used correctly the treatment cannot fail to produce the desired result. If this were not so the Chinese doctors could not have been as successful as they were.

FUNGI

Fungi, or yeasts, are believed to form part of the normal intestinal flora. The most common of these yeasts is Candida Albicans or Candida for short. We hear more about Candida than any other yeast because it is believed to cause the most trouble.

Since yeasts are so common, and they are found in everyone's digestive tract, how do we know that they are harmful? When they were first discovered it was believed that yeasts played a useful part in digestion and it was not suspected they could cause problems. When it became common knowledge that many symptoms can be alleviated by reducing the intake of refined carbohydrates (sugar, white flour, etc.) it was suggested that this happened partly because refined carbohydrates cause yeasts to proliferate excessively. This belief was strengthened even more when drugs, the best known of these is Nystantin, began to be used to control yeasts. The use of these drugs often produces such marked improvements that many symptoms are now believed to be caused by yeasts. The list is endless, ranging from fatigue, headaches and back pain to arthritis and various infections.

As a result of these findings it is now believed that as long as the immune system is strong, the body can prevent a yeast overgrowth. The yeasts remain in the digestive tract and not only do no harm but are believed to be useful in helping digestion and assimilation. If the body becomes rundown and weak the yeasts may proliferate excessively and invade other parts of the body. This happens most readily if refined carbohydrates are overindulged in. Refined carbohydrates are bad for the body and weaken it, while they promote rapid growth of the yeasts.

An interesting discovery has also been made

concerning the possible relationship of fungi to cancer. When the homeopathic imprinter, which kills a far wider spectrum of yeasts then drugs, began to be used for controlling fungi it was found that it is not unusual for so-called cancerous tumors to disappear when the homeopathic imprinter is used regularly. Presumably, fungal growths can be easily misdiagnosed as being cancerous tumors.

HOW THE HOMEOPATHIC IMPRINTER WORKS

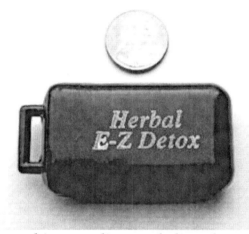

Homeopathic remedies are believed to produce their results by overpowering and killing bacteria and viruses with the enormously magnified vibrations these remedies emit.

As already briefly explained previously, a homeopathic remedy is made by placing a person's hand on the INPUT plate of the imprinter and the remedy (which is in a sealed plastic box-EZ Detox) on the OUTPUT plate. When this is done the remedy is imprinted with the greatly magnified vibrations in the person's hand. The patient's hand is then placed on the OUTPUT plate and the imprinted remedy on the INPUT plate. The imprinter then magnifies the vibrations in the remedy even more and imprints them back on the person's hand. When the tremendously magnified vibrations spread back through the patient's body they immediately clear it of all infections, parasites, Candida and many chemicals. All this takes only two or three seconds.

Once again, it is important to remember that the vibrations imprinted on the remedy are magnified many thousands of times by the imprinter.

Unless the remedy is damaged by water, moisture or by being placed in a strong magnetic field, it will retain the tremendously magnified vibrations indefinitely. It will be just as effective after a year, ten years or even a lot longer.

As already explained, the hand contains the vibrations of everything in the body; viruses, bacteria, parasites, chemicals, etc.. Therefore, as the enormously magnified vibrations emanating from the remedy pass through the body they clear it of everything that is imprinted on the remedy.

However, the remedy does nothing to reduce the tremendously damaging effects of dental restorations or jewelry which may contain such highly toxic metals as nickel or mercury. These metals have to be neutralized or removed by using the laser.

The homeopathic remedy also does nothing to remove metabolic waste from the body. The best way to do this is with the ionic foot bath when used together with the Metatron Electrical Energizer. These devices are described more fully in a later chapter. (When using the foot bath and the energizer you should not have the homeopathic remedy in your pocket. The electricity will immediately erase the vibrations imprinted on the remedy and make it ineffective).

If the plastic box, which contains the remedy, is kept on a person's body, in a pocket or tied around the neck, its vibrations will instantly spread to all parts of his body and keep it free of all the infections, parasites and chemicals whose vibrations are already imprinted on the remedy. But the homeopathic remedy will do nothing to remove viruses, bacteria, parasites or chemicals whose vibrations are not imprinted on it. Therefore, for best results, you should imprint the remedy after every meal or even more often. When you have done this always put the remedy in your pocket or anywhere on your body. Since it is impossible to tell when you might pick up something which has harmful vibrations, that are not yet imprinted on the remedy, you should use the imprinter as often as you can. You can only use it too little, never too much.

Amazingly, although the imprinter kills bad bacteria it does not affect the good bacteria in our gut. Unlike antibiotics, which can cause all kinds of problems by killing the friendly bacteria in our intestines, homeopathic remedies do not affect the friendly bacteria in any way.

The same applies to chemicals. The vibrations given off by the remedy either neutralize or remove chemicals in the same way that they kill bacteria and viruses. It is important to remember that at any time we may pick up new harmful vibrations from something that has not yet been imprinted on the remedy. It is therefore essential to use the imprinter frequently. After every meal or even more often. It only takes a few seconds to use the imprinter. After the remedy has been imprinted it should immediately be put in a pocket or somewhere on the body. YOU MUST CARRY THE REMEDY ON YOU ALL THE TIME.

WARNING

Homeopathic remedies immediately stop working if they become contaminated to the least degree. Unfortunately, this also applies to the homeopathic imprinter. Therefore, both the imprinter and the remedy have to be kept spotlessly clean. You have to wash your hands every time before using the imprinter.

To prevent contamination the imprinter has to be kept

in a plastic bag which must never be taken off. The homeopathic remedy box must also be kept in a plastic bag. These plastic bags should be changed at least every three days. In case of a more serious infection they should be changed every day to make sure there is no contamination causing interference. The easiest way to remove contamination is to laser the remedy and the imprinter for a few seconds every day. That is if you have a laser. If you have no laser, you can use a quartz crystal. Hold the crystal in one hand and the imprinter in the other. Then scan the box from all sides with crystal. If you don't hold the imprinter in your hand the crystal will do nothing. You have to pick up the vibrations of the imprinter by holding it in your hand. Then point the crystal at the imprinter from all sides. This will immediately neutralize any contaminants so they will no longer interfere.

SUMMARY

If you want to remain well you simply HAVE TO get your own homeopathic imprinter and use it after every meal. Infections and chemicals are the most frequent cause of symptoms such as headaches, fatigue, abdominal, chest, and mid-back pains, etc. so if you do not have an imprinter of your own you may have continual problems. The first step towards lasting health is to get your own imprinter. It is impossible to remain well for any length of time if you don't have your own imprinter and use it several times a day. Remember that just feeling well may not mean that nothing is wrong. Infections and chemicals do not always produce immediate symptoms. All that you may experience is more fatigue than usual, more headaches or pains and aches which you will not associate with a chronic, sub clinical infection or with chemical contamination.

The imprinter and the remedy will stop working immediately if they become contaminated. They have to be kept perfectly clean. IF YOU WANT TO STAY WELL THE MOST IMPORTANT SINGLE THING THAT YOU HAVE TO DO IS USE THE HOMEOPATHIC IMPRINTER CORRECTLY. You should read this chapter several times and make certain that you understand everything well. When you buy the imprinter you will be given a short CD which explains how it has to be used. The easiest way of keeping the imprinter working is to scan it with a quartz crystal before use. Such a crystal neutralizes any contamination which is preventing the imprinter from working. If possible you should buy a small hand held laser, the Q 1000 is by far the best choice.

CHAPTER 8
⌘
ENERGY FLOW BLOCKAGE

As has already been explained, in Eastern Medicine Chinese doctors believed that the only cause of all health problems is interference with the energy flow in the body. They found that if there is no interference sickness is impossible. The doctor's main job was to diagnose what was interfering with energy flow in his patient's body and remove the interference before the patient had any symptoms indicating that something was going wrong. If the doctor could do this successfully his patient would remain well and the doctor would get paid his usual fee, if the patient became sick that meant that the doctor had not removed the interference in time.

Therefore, it was the doctor's fault that the patient was sick. Consequently, to make up for his negligence, the doctor would have to treat the patient for free until he was well again.

In our Western Culture interference with the energy flow in the body is not recognized as a cause of health problems. Modern scientific discoveries have been so impressive that the methods used by Eastern Medicine have been looked down upon as outdated and primitive. Quite logically, it seemed to be impossible that there could be anything of real value in methods which were unscientific and already thousands of years old. Our modern scientific procedures had to be a lot better. As a result, our western diagnostic methods depend on such scientific procedures as: lab tests, blood tests, X-rays, MRIs and other modern technologies.

Quite obviously, if you think about it, none of our

scientific, modern methods do anything to improve the energy flow in the body or to help us discover what is interfering with the energy flow in a patient's body. In fact, the modern procedures we use often cause even more interference with the energy flow in the patient's body. The worst of these are probably drugs, radiation, chemotherapy and surgery.

It seems logical to assume that our failure to recognize the importance of interference with the energy flow in the body is the main and often the only reason why we can do nothing to help chronic conditions. Since chronic conditions are caused entirely by interference with the energy flow in the body, drugs and surgery and other modern procedures can do no more than mask symptoms, while the condition or problem gradually gets worse and worse.

Until the importance of the energy flow in the body is recognized and understood no satisfactory solution to chronic health problems can ever or will ever be found. Conversely, once it is recognized that chronic conditions are caused by interference with the energy flow in the body it will become very easy to prevent or even cure them.

I am a perfect example of what happens when our modern methods are tried. As long as these methods were used I kept being told that my case was hopeless and that there was nothing that anyone could do for me. It was just a matter of how long I could still live, a day, a week or possibly even another month. When the eastern approach was tried and the energy flow in my body improved I immediately felt at least fifty percent better and I have been improving ever since.

The treatments that were used on me previously only made me worse. I became badly bloated and I gained over sixty pounds. When I stopped these treatments (drugs) I not only began improving steadily but I have also dropped a lot of weight. I am now over sixty pounds lighter and all my friends keep telling me how healthy and fit I look. I spend an hour and a half every day in the gym trying to regain my fitness; this is something I could not possibly have done if I was having the treatments recommended for cancer.

The same thing happened to Dolores Geisler. As long as she continued being treated with western methods the cancer kept coming back and Dolores kept getting sicker. The drugs and steroids made her gain a hundred and twenty pounds and when the cancer came back for the fourth time she was told that she was terminal and there was no longer anything anybody could do for her. When the eastern approach was tried and all the factors that were interfering with the energy flow in her body were removed, Dolores began improving at once and within a short time her cancer was gone and has never come back.

I have since spoken to many people who suffered from incurable chronic conditions which our western methods could do nothing for. These people also often began getting better when the new methods were used on them. Once the causes of interference with the energy flow in their bodies were removed they soon improved. In many cases all their symptoms cleared up and they were able to enjoy a level of health they had never thought possible. The problems they had were such chronic conditions as: rheumatoid arthritis, fibromyalgia, M.S. (multiple sclerosis), paralysis, crippling back pains, cataracts, poor vision, heart problems, C.F.S. (chronic fatigue syndrome), infections (for which the only cure was amputation), asthma, disabling allergies, scoliosis, life threatening osteoporosis, terrible skin conditions for which there appeared to be no cure, disfiguring psoriasis, life threatening infections and other problems. It seems that there is nothing that cannot be helped if treatment can be started in time and all the reasons for interference with the energy flow in the body are removed.

FROM ALL THIS IT IS CLEAR THAT CHRONIC CONDITIONS ARE THE RESULT OF CHRONIC INTERFERENCE WITH THE ENERGY FLOW IN OUR BODIES. THEREFORE, THE ONLY WAY THAT A CHRONIC CONDITION CAN BE PREVENTED OR TREATED IS BY REMOVING ALL THE FACTORS WHICH ARE CAUSING INTERFERENCE WITH THE ENERGY FLOW.

The problem has been that the eastern methods of diagnosing what is interfering with the energy flow in a patient's body are so vague and difficult to understand that it is very difficult for us to learn them. As a result, in spite of the obviously remarkable successes of the eastern approach to illness, no organized effort has ever been made to discover exactly how eastern medicine works.

The first Western doctors to take a serious interest in the eastern methods were the European homeopaths who use electro-diagnosis. These doctors made a discovery of tremendous importance. They found that the energy flow in the body is very strongly affected and improves enormously (among other things causing weak muscles to become a lot stronger) if a homeopathic remedy or a nutritional supplement that the body is lacking or needs is placed on the skin.

For instance, if a vitamin or mineral or some other nutritional supplement that a person needs or lacks is placed in close contact with their skin there is an immediate huge improvement in the energy flow in their body. This then results in a general relaxation and realignment of the entire body. It also causes an amazing increase in the strength of weak muscles. The difference is not very slight and difficult to detect, it is enormous and easy to measure.

The best and easiest way to detect the body's reactions is to use the method shown in the following diagrams. Since it has been found that the energy flow is also affected by colors or even colored objects that a person happens to be wearing, or looking at, to prevent errors the individual who is being tested has to be covered with a white sheet (it is believed that the colors white and black are neutral and do not affect the energy flow) and the patient has to close his eyes to prevent him from looking at any colored objects.

In the first illustration it can be seen that if a person lies on their stomach and their legs are raised there will be a considerable difference in the height of the legs when the legs are firmly pressed down. If no pressure is used the legs may be even, but when firm pressure is applied the weaker leg will not be able to resist as well and it will "give", causing it to appear shorter or lower.

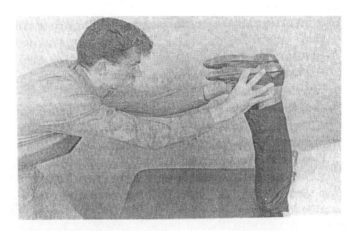

Illustration 1 This photo shows a person being checked for a difference in the height of their legs. In most cases an easily detectable difference can be found. Often, if enough pressure is applied, the difference can be as much as one inch. It is important to cover the person who is being tested with a white sheet because the colors of clothing can affect the test. White and black are neutral colors and do not appear to affect the test. Bright colors (blue, red, yellow, etc) can make the test

invalid. This method is so simple that if you have strong hands, and a little training, you could easily use it in your home to determine the causes of simple conditions.

The second illustration shows how the legs immediately even out, due to the instant increase in the strength of the muscles of the weaker leg, if anything that improves the energy flow is placed on the person's back. For instance, if a vitamin B 12 tablet is placed on the person's back nothing will happen (and the legs will remain uneven) if there is no deficiency in B12 and the patient does not need it. If he does have a deficiency of B12, placing the B12 on his back will cause an immediate huge improvement in the energy flow in his body and the legs will even out at once and they cannot be made to become uneven again no matter how much pressure is used. More vitamin B12 tablets can then be added until the amount the person needs is reached. When too much of the B12 is placed on the person's back this will again cause interference with the energy flow and the legs will become uneven again. This method, therefore, makes it possible to discover not only what deficiencies are present but also exactly how much of any supplement a person may need at any given time.

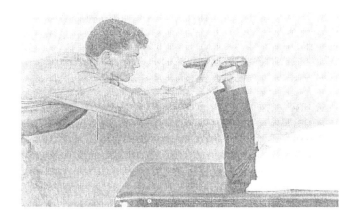

Illustration 2 Here the subject is being tested for a deficiency of thiamin (vitamin B1). It can be seen that the legs have evened out, indicating that he lacks thiamin. This is a very important vitamin and its lack can cause many symptoms, such as: headaches, depression, inability to concentrate. The person doing the testing should also wear neutral colors and no metals---watches, rings, any jewelry.

By using homeopathic remedies the same procedure can also be used to determine what else is wrong. For instance, if a homeopathic remedy for Staff bacteria is placed on the patient's back and this causes the legs to even out, that means that the patient has a Staff infection. If the homeopathic imprinter is used the new way this will immediately kill the Staff bacteria and the patient's body will no longer react to the homeopathic remedy for Staff.

There are homeopathic remedies for every condition. If this method is used correctly it is possible to discover, in just a few minutes, what is wrong with a patient. What deficiencies are present, what allergies a person may have, what infections, what organ weaknesses, etc. In many cases this method of diagnosis is infinitely better, quicker and less costly than anything ever discovered in the past. Since the body makes no mistakes, errors in diagnosis cannot be made if everything is done correctly.

The easiest way to check for weakness or malfunction of the organs is to use the supplements produced by Standard Process. This company's supplements are specifically made for each organ: the heart, lungs, liver, adrenal glands, etc. Placing these supplements on a person's back is an excellent way of determining what organ weaknesses are present.

European doctors believe that with the new discoveries we could now not only easily prevent cancer but also practically all of the other chronic health problems which cause such misery in our lives and for which, so far, we have been quite unable to find any satisfactory solutions.

Some of the factors that the Chinese were known to consider as being important in causing interference with the energy flow in the body were: unfitness, poor posture, nutritional deficiencies, infections, intestinal parasites and harmful emotions.

More recently homeopaths discovered a number of other factors which can also play an important part in blocking the energy flow. These factors include: scars, calluses, allergies, dental restorations made of toxic and harmful metals, the misalignment produced by the head shifting off center on the spine (see CH. 12), chemicals, many items of jewelry, heavy metal toxicity and toxicity due to poor elimination of metabolic waste.

When the new method of diagnosis is used it is possible to find many problems which were entirely overlooked in the past. For instance, this method has shown that virtually everyone's body is contaminated with aluminum, lead, nickel, mercury, pesticides and numerous other chemicals. Since mercury in dental fillings cause thyroid weakness practically everyone has hypothyroidism. Almost everyone is also found to have intestinal parasites and a large number have undiagnosed, sub clinical infections.

Since many of the diagnostics and drugs used by modern medicine are ineffective for detecting or correcting these problems it is not surprising that we now have more sickness than ever before.

SUMMARY

If you have an accident or other serious emergency you have to go to the hospital to be treated. You have no choice. Hospitals are the only places that have the necessary equipment to deal with catastrophic situations.

But if you have a chronic condition and there is no immediate danger to your life, then taking drugs, to cover up your symptoms, will not help. If you want to get well you have to somehow find a doctor who uses the methods described in this book. Unless the method of diagnosis shown in the diagrams in this chapter is used it is very costly, difficult or impossible for anyone to determine what is causing your problems. This method is the only way to discover what is interfering with the energy flow in your body. If the interference with the energy flow is not removed it is impossible to correct chronic health problems.

When other methods of diagnoses are used they cannot possibly help us discover what is causing interference with the energy flow.

Once again, no matter how good your doctor may be he cannot truly help you unless you learn how to do as many things as possible for yourself.

Drugs are so toxic and cause so much interference with the energy flow that if you keep taking drugs it may be impossible to restore the energy flow in your body back to normal. Just about the worst in this respect are probably such powerful pain killers as morphine, methadone and Oxycontin. If you want to get well and stay well you have to ask your doctor how you could get off drugs, as soon as possible. Stopping drugs cold turkey can be dangerous.

Other methods of diagnosis may have some limited value, but unless the method of diagnosis explained in this chapter is used most health problems can be badly misdiagnosed.

Some doctors in Europe even believe that most breast cancers in women are caused by the under wires in bras. This is because under wires are made out of an alloy which contains nickel. Nickel is carcinogenic and is used to cause tumors in experimental animals. The only way to neutralize or remove the nickel is with a low level laser. You must somehow find a doctor who has such a laser or buy your own and put your bra and jewelry under it.

CHAPTER 9

⌘

CLEANSING

One of the main reasons why we have been so unsuccessful in helping people with chronic conditions is because so little is done to cleanse patients' bodies of parasites, chemicals and metabolic wastes.

A good example is cancer. As already explained earlier in the book, it is believed in Europe that cancer is nothing but a symptom that the body is drowning in a sea of pollution. If the body can be cleansed in time, the cancer can reverse and go away. Holistic doctors believe that cancer will not exist if the body is not toxic and the immune system is strong.

Heart trouble is another good example. In most people heart trouble is nothing more than a symptom that the body needs cleansing. If you don't believe this consider how quickly patients recover from even very serious heart problems when natural cleansing methods are used. For instance, at the, Weimar Institute New Start Program, a Seventh Day Adventist facility in Weimar, California, patients with heart problems are placed on fresh juices and a strict program of natural cleansing foods. They also go for long walks in the woods and spend time every day in saunas and having massages. When this is done, often in a few weeks the cholesterol plaque in the heart arteries is cleared out and the patients' health improves dramatically. Even many patients with ninety percent occlusions (blockages of the arteries) have recovered rapidly when this approach was used. They no longer needed bypass surgery and they could stop taking drugs. One doctor whom I spoke to even said that, "ninety-seven percent of heart surgeries are unnecessary".

Fibromyalgia is another good example. This condition responds so well to cleansing that patients often recover in a short time. When drugs are used victims suffer endlessly, without any hope of recovery.

CFS (chronic fatigue syndrome) patients frequently recover readily when their bodies are cleansed. Drugs are useless for this condition and patients often continue to suffer indefinitely.

Acne and many other skin conditions also often clear up readily when patients cleanse their bodies. Drugs, at best, give relief from itching or reduce inflammation, while causing the body to become even more toxic.

Other conditions which respond well to cleansing are: Type II Diabetes, joint pains, obesity, fatigue, osteoporosis, headaches and numerous other problems.

If instead of drugs natural cleansing methods were used---together with the laser, the ionic foot bath, the Metatron Electrical Energizer and the imprinter---there would be new hope for many of the people who are suffering from chronic conditions for which there was little hope in the past.

THE IONIC FOOT BATH

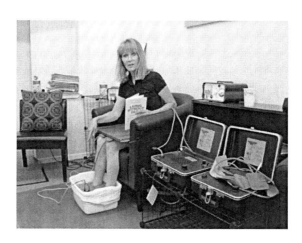

When used together the ionic foot bath and the Metatron Electrical Energizer are probably the best and fastest way of cleansing the body discovered so far. The ionic foot bath gets its name from the fact that an ionizing unit is placed in the water of the foot bath. This ionizer then splits the water into oxygen and hydrogen gases, or ions. These oxygen and hydrogen ions then penetrate through the skin and are carried to all parts of the body where they combine with organic waste and oxidize it.

The oxidized waste then passes back through the skin and into the water in the foot bath. Everyone should use the ionic foot bath at least once a week to prevent the body from becoming too toxic. Apart from helping in the removal of wastes the ionic foot bath may also reduce swelling and inflammation, not just in the feet but in the entire body. It also helps remove calluses, improve circulation and promote healing.

THE METATRON ELECTRICAL ENERGIZER

The Metatron Electrical Energizer is a form of electrical stimulation whose purpose is to help the body heal faster. It has been found that if the foot bath is used together with the Energizer it will draw far more waste out of the body than if the footbath is used alone. When used together the Energizer and the foot bath have also been found to speed up healing tremendously. Some people believe that in some cases the Energizer may speed up healing by as much as five to ten times. There have been cases where wounds and other damage to tissues which healed sluggishly, or in some cases would not heal at all following injuries, began healing again when the foot bath and the Energizer were used together.

NUTRITION SUCCESSES

There is overwhelming evidence that cancer is not a disease in itself but only a symptom that the body has become overloaded with toxic wastes. This is the opinion of holistic doctors and researchers   For instance, in his book "The Cancer Prevention Diet," Michio Kushi writes, "Cancer is the terminal stage of a long process. Cancer is the body's healthy attempt to isolate toxins ingested and accumulated through years of eating the modern unnatural diet and living in an artificial environment. Cancer is the body's last drastic effort to prolong life, even for a few more years. By gathering the unwanted materials in local areas, the rest of the body is maintained in a relatively clean and functioning condition. This process of localization is part of our natural healing power, saving us from total breakdown."

"But the modern view looks upon these localizations as dangerous enemies which have to be destroyed and removed. Its attitude can be compared to the behavior of a city troubled by too much waste. Instead of investigating the source of the waste and helping the sanitation department to deal with the problem more effectively, the city tries to destroy the waste by using measures that not only make the situation a lot worse, by creating more waste, but also weaken the sanitation department and make it a lot more difficult, or even impossible, for it to do its job."

In his book, <u>A Cancer Therapy, Results of Fifty Cases,</u> Dr. Max Gerson quotes fifty cases of terminal cancer patients who recovered when their bodies were cleansed with fresh juices and coffee enemas. All these people would have most certainly died, or they would have been severely crippled for life, if they had continued having the conventional, scientific treatments used for killing tumors and cancer cells.

In her book <u>The Grape Fast</u>, Johanna Huss explains

how she cured even the worst cases of cancer by placing patients on a diet consisting of nothing but fresh, ripe seeded red grapes. In Spain certain clinics give cancer patients only ripe peaches and tumors disappear so fast that a huge improvement often occurs from one day to the next.

The problem is that science does not want to admit to the validity of all this evidence and conveniently labels these natural cancer cures as "spontaneous remissions" or "misdiagnoses". Admitting that cancer is only a symptom of toxicity and that it can be cured with simple natural methods for cleansing the body would put an end to very attractive research grants and it would also cause catastrophic losses to the cancer industry. All those millions generated by surgeries, chemotherapy and radiation therapy would suddenly disappear into thin air. Instead they would be replaced with such unattractive things as machines for making fresh juices and equipment for doing colonics.

RADIATION POISONING

There is no money in natural methods, but financial rewards for prescribing chemotherapy and radiation are astronomical.

Radiation poisoning is now so common that it is becoming a leading cause of many health problems, especially cancer. One of the leading hospitals in California recently reported that they had FORTY times more cases of brain tumors that ever before, due to the use of cell phones and other electronic devices.

Getting rid of radiation poisoning is now easy. All you have to do is place a homeopathic remedy for radiation on the INPUT plate of the homeopathic imprinter and your fingers on the OUTPUT plate. When you activate the imprinter it will imprint your fingers with the radiation vibrations and when these enormously magnified vibrations pass through your body they immediately neutralize the radiation vibrations which have been harming your body.

This simple procedure is producing amazing results. Some patients with very serious conditions have spontaneously improved or even recovered. For instance, in one case a young girl's legs became paralyzed. She spent over a month in the hospital's I.C.U., had every possible treatment used on her without success. No reason for the paralysis could be determined. When the radiation was removed from her body, by using the simple method explained above, she recovered almost immediately and has had no further problems.

In another case a middle aged man developed what was diagnosed as Parkinson's disease. He lost the use of his right hand and leg. When the radiation was removed from his body he immediately regained full use of his leg and his hand also improved.

CELLUAR PHONES

Cellular phone use emits dangerous vibrations right into the ear canal and seems to be causing an epidemic of cancerous brain tumors. Recently, a local hospital reported a twenty-fold (or 2,000%) increase in the incidence of malignancies of the brain. It recently came out in National TV News that cellular phone use has definitely been linked to brain cancer. Kinesiology testing shows that this is due to the cancer causing effect of mercury being somehow increased enormously by the use of cellular phones. Unless a cancer patient stops cellular phone use altogether, it may impede recovery. This puts cellular phone use in the extremely dangerous category. It seems to create "super toxic" mercury which causes tumors to grow at a record pace.

FUNGI, MOLDS AND YEASTS

You can get rid of these parasites in a similar way to radiation poisoning. Just place a homeopathic remedy for fungi, yeasts, and molds on the INPUT plate of the imprinter and your fingers on the OUTPUT plate. When you activate the imprinter the enormously magnified vibrations of yeasts, molds, and fungi will pass through your tissues and clear your body. If you can repeat this procedure enough times, after a few months you may find that even your nail fungus is gone, a good indicator that the fungus is cleared in your entire body.

CHAPTER 10

⌘

SCARS AND CALLUSES

As previously explained, in Eastern Medicine Chinese doctors found that as long as the energy flow in the body is not interfered with in any way a patient remains healthy.

Unless they are treated every day scars cause massive interference with the energy flow in our bodies, no matter how small or old they may be. They play an important part in causing all health problems, although in most cases we are quite unaware of the tremendously damaging effects caused by scars.

It has recently been discovered that scars always cause weakness of the muscles of one side of the body. In some individuals the difference is so great that the muscles of one side of the body may appear to be as much as five or even ten times as strong or weak as those of the other side. Even the smallest scars always cause a significant difference.

The interference with the energy flow caused by scars results in the body becoming unstable, because of the differences in the strength of the muscles. It is an important cause of osteo-arthritis or degenerative arthritis of the joints. This is the name given to the wearing out or degeneration of the joints of the spine, hips and knees. Osteo arthritis often plays an important part in causing pain and other serious problems in older people. It is the main cause of back surgeries, hip surgeries and knee surgeries. If the scars are treated, they no longer interfere with the flow of energy in the body and the difference in muscle strength immediately disappears. The two sides become equally strong. If you treat your scars daily there will soon be a significant improvement, whether you are conscious of this or not. Your muscles will be stronger, your organs and everything in your body will function better.

Another important problem that has been discovered is that scars, no matter how small or how few, always cause a sensitivity or allergy to such important nutrients as proteins, carbohydrates, calcium and many other essential foods. This can then result in a host of problems such as fatigue, difficulty concentrating, weakness, and cavities in the teeth, osteoporosis, dry skin and many others. When the scars are treated, that is to say firmly rubbed with vitamin E and A oil, all these sensitivities cease at once. You will get even better results if you can also use a hand held laser for treating both your scars and your entire body. They help to deepen the healing and reduce the painful adhesions associated with many surgical scars.

CALLUSES

In many cases calluses and dry thickened skin on the feet cause more trouble and more interference with energy flow than scars. To correct this problem the calluses and dry skin have to be treated every day. First, they must be taken off by using a pumice stone and then the skin has to be rubbed firmly with vitamin A & E oil to soften it up and improve the energy flow.

Treating the calluses and any dry skin on the feet this way has produced remarkable results in many individuals. Some of the symptoms that have improved, or even gone away, include: chronic back pain, fatigue, headaches, dry skin and many others.

SUMMARY

If you want to enjoy good health you have to treat your scars daily by rubbing them firmly with vitamin A and E oil and, if possible by also using a hand held laser on them at least once or twice a day. If you do not do this you will have more and more trouble as the years pass. Scars have an absolutely devastating effect on the energy flow in the body and on our health. Don't ask a professional person whether this is true or not, it is almost certain that he will know nothing about the harmful effects of scars.

But don't forget that tattoos, piercings, stretch marks, calluses and areas of thickened dry skin (above all on the feet) have the same effect as scars. They all block the energy flow. This is especially true of calluses. They cause more interference with the energy flow than almost anything else.

Drugs are some of the worst poisons; they can really make cleansing efforts extremely difficult. If a sick person is on heavy pain medication, or they are using other drugs, it may be impossible to cleanse their body sufficiently. If that is the case the methods explained in this book may not work. Drugs are such vile poisons and they interfere to such a degree with normal metabolism that they may make recovery impossible. Ask your doctors how you can get off the medications you are taking.

CHAPTER 11
✼
ALLERGIES

About 15 years ago Dr. Devi Nambudripad, a California Acupuncturist, Chiropractor and Kinesiologist made what is perhaps the most important discovery ever made concerning allergies. She found that by tapping up and down the middle of a patient's back, while the patient is holding or touching something he is allergic to, she could reprogram the body's response to the allergen in such a way that it would no longer recognize it as being harmful.

By using this simple method it is now possible to desensitize oneself to anything that one is allergic to. The result is that in a matter of just a few minutes you are no longer allergic to things you were allergic to before and they no longer cause you any problems.

This method produces such amazing results that Dr. Nambudripad wrote several books in which she quotes numerous testimonials from persons who experienced truly miraculous recoveries when this technique was used on them. This desensitization method, known as NAET, has now become so popular that it is used all over the world. The procedure has even been recognized by the FDA and is covered by insurance companies.

The results produced by this simple method have been so outstanding that Dr Nambudripad has written several books with such titles as: Say Good Bye to Illness, Say Good Bye to ADD and ADHD, Living Pain Free, Say Goodbye to Autism and several others.

The results produced by NAET have been truly amazing. For instance, Dr. Nambudripad quotes the story of a man whose hand became "frozen in a clenched position" following an accident. He could not use it for three years and he was in constant pain. After only a few sessions with this method, the man regained full use of his hand, had no pain and was able to go back to work. When this patient was desensitized to different allergens his condition, which appeared to have nothing to do with allergies, resolved itself.

Another man was so sensitive to oranges that if he ate anything that contained even the smallest amount of orange he would go into a coma and had to be rushed to the hospital by ambulance. When he held an orange in his hand and the doctor used the allergy desensitization method, the allergy stopped at once and oranges no longer caused him any trouble. In another case, a woman was so allergic to her cats that she had serious problems if one of them even came close to her. When she held some of the cat hair in her hand and she was desensitized the allergy stopped immediately. From that moment on she had no more trouble and she could kiss, hug and stroke her cats.

Recently, a discovery has been made which makes this allergy desensitization method even easier and faster to use. It has been found that all you have to do to reprogram your body's response to allergens is to hold or touch the offending substance and tap firmly up and down the middle of your chest with the other hand or fist. You can do this in the privacy of your home or at any time. It costs you nothing and only takes a few seconds. If you tap too gently nothing will happen.

Even better, it has been found that you do not have to desensitize yourself to one thing at a time, as was originally believed to be necessary. You can desensitize yourself to any number of different allergens at the same time. As a result, a small box has now been prepared which contains literally thousands of different substances which are known to cause allergic symptoms. If you hold this box in one hand and tap firmly up and down the middle of your chest with the fist of your other hand you can desensitize yourself to all these common allergens at the same time. It only takes a few seconds and does not cost a dime.

The following is a quote from a letter written by a person who used this method: "I have had allergies for as long as I can remember. I am now fifty-five. The allergies caused me a runny nose, itchy eyes, extreme fatigue, difficulty concentrating, irritability, difficulty in getting along with others, terrible night sweats and depression. When I began using the allergy desensitization box all these symptoms stopped at once. If they start again I immediately tap up and down the middle of my chest while holding the box in my other hand and the symptoms stop within a few minutes. The medications I had taken previously also stopped the symptoms, but they used to give me sinus headaches and pressure, while the decongestants caused me to feel as if swarms of ants were crawling all over my body."

THE CAUSES OF ALLERGIES

It will probably never be understood exactly why one person is allergic to something while another person in not allergic to the same thing. We will also probably never understand the exact mechanism which triggers allergic reactions, but so far two definite causes of allergies have been found. These are scars and general toxicity of the body. It is now known that scars, tattoos, piercings, calluses, scratches and skin abrasions of any kind immediately cause sensitivity to such common nutrients as vitamins, proteins, carbohydrates and others. These allergies or sensitivities then cause devastating problems which may literally wreck our lives. The patient himself usually has no idea what is happening and tries to control his symptoms with decongestants or other medications.

There is no doubt that the harm that scars cause is due to the scar tissue blocking the surface energy flow in the body. The Chinese acupuncture meridians, which carry energy to all parts of the body, run near the surface of the skin. By using needles inserted in strategic points, Chinese doctors balance the energy in the body and relieve many health problems. If the scars are softened, by being rubbed firmly with vitamin A and E oil, the flow of energy along the meridians improves at once and truly miraculous changes immediately take place, whether you actually notice anything or not. Muscles become stronger and the allergies to basic nutrients immediately disappear. The results are so incredible that it is obvious that to remain healthy everyone should make a point of rubbing their scars vigorously every day.

One of the most amazing recoveries occurred in a man who had a bad fall when he was twelve years old. For the next forty-nine years he had constant pain in his left shoulder and he had lost the use of his left arm during the last seven years. When his scars were rubbed he immediately regained the use of his arm and the pain stopped for the first time in 42 years.

In another case, a woman who had a tic (involuntary twitching of the facial muscles) found that as long as she rubbed a small scar on the calf of her leg the tic did not come back.

FOOD ALLERGIES

Although it is true that we can now desensitize ourselves to foods we are allergic to, this does not mean that it is good for us to eat highly processed, unnatural foods. It is clearly impossible to entirely remove the harmful effects of these foods. In his book Don't Settle for a Migraine Headache,

Dr. George Malcolm writes, "Two of my patients, a musician age 24 and a farmer age 36 were found to be sensitive to cheese. When this single item was eliminated from their diets, both lost over forty pounds and their lower back pain stopped."

From the above example, it is clear that it is difficult to enjoy truly good health if one eats cheese, biscuits made of white refined flour, white bread or any other highly refined, unnatural foods which have been radically changed by processing. Packaged foods usually contain rancid oils, chemical additives and preservatives and have terrible food combining properties.

The following is a list of foods which many test subjects were found to be sensitive to. If you want to enjoy good health you should not eat these:

- All nuts, except almonds. It appears likely that the fat content in most nuts such as cashews, sunflower seeds or peanuts is so high that they easily go rancid soon after being shelled. If fresh they are all good.
- Fruit skins, with the exception of fruits with very delicate skins such as cherries, cherry tomatoes and some grapes.
- All unripe fruit. It is surprising to find that the two halves of the same apple or pear can produce opposite effects. The half that is ripe causes no reaction, while the half that is not ripe causes a negative reaction.
- Iceberg lettuce
- Many brands of chewing gum
- Many brands of soft drinks
- Most tap water and some brands of bottled water
- Most breads
- Bananas. The reason for this is hard to understand. Perhaps the starch in the fruit is changed by storage.

- Most brands of granola, protein powders and other powdered foods. These foods oxidize rapidly after being processed soon becomes rancid. When fresh they are okay.
- Oils and fats if they are rancid
- Some deodorants, lipsticks, hair sprays and cosmetics
- Pasteurized and homogenized milk products
- Foods containing refined sugar
- Most drugs
- Tea, coffee, alcoholic beverages, bottled and canned juices
- Some meats, spices and dressings
- Many dried fruits

The following is a list of foods which are seldom found to cause problems:

- Untreated, raw almonds. This is probably due to their low fat content
- Most fruits when pealed
- Romaine lettuce
- Most vegetables whether raw or lightly cooked
- Some honeys. Honey may be polluted with chemicals
- Distilled water and some bottled waters
- Fresh whole grain foods
- Bread made with sour dough, not yeast. The flour that bread is made of has to be freshly ground. It rapidly goes rancid.
- Fresh, raw untreated milk, fresh butter made out of unpasteurized milk.

In short the rule seems to be: don't eat foods which have been changed and damaged by man. Try to eat only those foods which are fresh and are as natural as possible.

ALLERGIC SYMPTOMS ARE NOT ALWAYS CAUSED BY ALLERGENS.

You will be surprised to know that allergic symptoms are not always caused by allergens. If one has such symptoms as sneezing, coughing, phlegm, asthma and other problems, we automatically assume that they are the symptoms of allergies. However, more often than not, such symptoms are not caused by allergies but by something else. Real allergic symptoms are frequently quite different. The symptoms that we commonly associate with allergies are usually caused either by chronic, sub-clinical infections, which could not be diagnosed with lab tests, or by a weakness of the heart, the adrenal glands or the thyroid. In most cases the chronic sub-clinical infections are the main cause. The reason this is not understood is because our modern diagnostic methods often cannot detect these mild infections and consequently the part they play in causing so called allergic symptoms is overlooked.

SUMMARY

You should somehow try to get the allergy box described in this chapter. Using it regularly, usually at least twice a day, will make a big difference, whether you notice it or not. You must also rub your scars with oil and use the imprinter regularly.

CHAPTER 12

⌘

SPINAL MISALIGNMENTS AND THE AMAZING HEALING POWER OF CRYSTALS

Until fairly recently, it was believed that true misalignments cannot occur in the spine. Medical doctors entirely disregarded the possibility that spinal misalignments could occur and play an important part in causing health problems, while osteopaths used only crude manipulative methods. The results were so poor and inconsistent that they were given little consideration. On the other hand, in the chiropractic profession it was assumed that back problems were chiefly the result of what was known as "fixations". This was the name given to areas of the back where free movement was restricted by muscles which for some reason could not or would not relax fully.

As a result, the main purpose of chiropractic treatments was to try and relax and mobilize these stiff, tight areas. This was done by using spinal manipulation and various other methods to try and get the contracted muscles to relax.

Once again the results were so poor and inconsistent that chiropractic adjustments were considered to be of little value.

Improvements in X-ray techniques have recently enabled us to take more accurate X-rays of the spine. Thanks to this it has finally been possible to demonstrate that a very damaging misalignment does in fact occur between the head and the atlas vertebra. The atlas is the name given to the vertebra that supports the head.

It is now known that as long as the head is centered on the atlas, so that there is no misalignment between the atlas and the skull, the entire body remains relaxed and well aligned. There can be no scoliosis (sideward curvature of the spine), the pelvis remains level and the legs are even when checked with the patient lying on his back.

However, if for some reason the head slips off center on the atlas, this then causes pressure on the brain stem which results in general involuntary contraction and spasm of the muscles of one side of the body. From the contraction the muscles cannot relax, as long as there is pressure on the brain stem by the misaligned atlas vertebra they will keep the entire body twisted at all times. Whether a person is moving, standing, sitting or lying. Because of this the pelvis becomes uneven and rotated and the legs and arms become uneven in length when checked with a person lying on their back.

Since the muscles can never relax fully, as long as there is pressure on the brain stem by the misaligned atlas, this exhausts the body terribly. The misalignment of the head on the atlas vertebra plays an important part in causing: nutritional deficiencies, osteo-arthritis, osteoporosis, cavities in the teeth, hormone problems, scoliosis, uneven development of muscles, etc., etc.

The misalignment of the head on the atlas results in so much interference with normal function that it plays an important part in causing all health problems. It would probably be no exaggeration to say that the misalignment of the atlas accounts for close to half of our health problems, especially when we get older.

For instance, it has been found that when the misalignment is corrected deficiencies of vitamins and minerals may drop by as much as ninety percent, or they may even disappear entirely. The misalignment of the head on the atlas is often the main cause of female problems: irregular periods, miscarriages, inability to conceive, and painful menstrual periods.

If you want to prevent health problems you absolutely have to try and find a good chiropractor who uses the NUCCA (NATIONAL UPPERCERVICAL CHIROPRACTIC ASSOCIATION) method for adjusting the atlas. Only the NUCCA method is truly accurate and only this method consistently gives wonderful results.

When the head is brought back to the exact center on the atlas the entire body relaxes and straightens out and there is a tremendous general improvement. The results are often nothing short of miraculous. Patients with just about every known condition have either improved or even recovered fully after this adjustment. This is because the patients' bodies were finally able to relax and function better. At the end of this section you will find the stories of several patients who only recovered when their atlas was finally adjusted back to center by using the precision NUCCA adjusting method. These stories will give you a better understanding of the tremendously damaging effects that the misalignment of the head on the spine can have on our health.

Precision adjusting of the atlas back to center under the head is unfortunately difficult and although it gives such wonderful results, it is still very hard to find a chiropractor who uses the new precision adjusting NUCCA method. A number of methods for adjusting the head back to center on the atlas have been developed but unfortunately they are all still very crude and inaccurate and do a very poor job. Only the NUCCA method is truly accurate and only this method consistently gives wonderful results.

Case history #1   This patient was involved in a major car accident. The car slipped on ice and rolled down an embankment. Her back and pelvis were broken. Surgery was performed and two nine inch rods were inserted on each side of the patient's spine. Metal plates were also used to hold her pelvis together. The patient was told that she would never walk again and she would have to use a wheelchair. When this patient's atlas was adjusted using the NUCCA precision adjusting method all her pain left. A month later she was able to go water skiing. She also uses a crystal to keep her skull aligned and she treats her scars daily with a laser and rubs them firmly with vitamin A and E oil.

Case history #2 This patient writes: "In 1982 I had an industrial accident that caused a compression fracture of my lower back (L5 S1 area). I was seen by several MDs including one of the finest neurosurgeons in the Pacific Northwest. In their opinion I could only live a very sedentary life and they warned that I could become a paraplegic at any time."

"With this cheerful diagnosis I prepared for a life of pain and inactivity. For the next twelve years that was indeed the way that my life progressed. I was in chronic pain with frequent bouts of acute pain that caused me to be bedridden for weeks at a time. This was all that the doctors could do except to recommend narcotic pain killers and fit me with a tens unit to try to manage the worst of the symptoms."

"In 1994 my fiancé suggested that I go to a NUCCA chiropractor to have my atlas and skull adjusted. She said that this had helped her a lot, while six months of spinal manipulation had given no relief. After only two atlas adjustments and a program of mineral supplements I have not only been pain free, but I have been able to practice martial arts. The traditional medical community had told me that my case was hopeless and two atlas adjustments cured me in two visits. I cannot express how grateful I am to have found this method. Thanks to it I now lead a life that I never dreamed would be possible."

Case history #3 This young girl writes: "In the spring of 2002 I slipped on some ice and injured my lower back. I was seen by a number of doctors all of whom eventually said that they had no idea what was wrong with me. The only thing that helped a little was physical therapy.

Since medicine seemed to have nothing to offer I decided to try chiropractic. The first chiropractor told me that my case was very serious and it would take him a whole year to correct all my misalignments. I had to see him three times a week for four months, twice a week for four months and then once a week for the last four months, a total of one hundred times. He used a so called activator to correct my misalignment.

When I was no better at the end of the year I began going to a second chiropractor. He also saw me a hundred times over the course of a year and used manual manipulation, which he said was much better than the activator. During every session I could hear all my bones crack and pop as my spine realigned itself. But at the end of the year I was a lot worse instead of better. The pain kept waking me up in the night, I could not run or take part in sports and the pain, fatigue and headaches interfered with my schooling and other activities. I began losing hope that I would ever get well again.

When a friend heard of the problems I was having, she suggested that I go and see her chiropractor who she said uses the NUCCA method. Because of the lack of success I had had with chiropractors, I was unwilling to go but she insisted and took me to her chiropractor's office. I could not believe it when after only one adjustment all my pain left at once. I have now been pain free for over a year."

If enough money was available for such a project, special centers should be organized where people could go to have their skull and atlas adjusted. If everyone was properly aligned and they were taught to do the back exercises and how to use the crystal, this would prevent endless problems. It would also save an untold amount of suffering and countless millions in unnecessary expenses.

MISALIGNMENTS OF THE
BONES OF THE HEAD

It has been known for a long time that the bones of the head (skull) can also misalign and these cranial (skull) misalignments may result in all kinds of problems, similar to those caused by the head misaligning on the atlas.

Consequently, if the adjustment of the head back to center on the atlas is to be effective, the skull itself has to be adjusted also.

The problem is that it is almost impossible to find anyone who knows how to go about adjusting the bones of the head. Some osteopaths and chiropractors will try to make you believe they know something but the bones of the head misalign again so easily that it may be difficult to obtain lasting results.

A wonderful solution to this problem has recently been discovered in the most unexpected way. Amazingly, it has been found that if a large quartz crystal (half a pound or more) is pointed at the different bones of the head the energy emanating from the crystal causes the misaligned bones in the head to realign themselves immediately. When this is done the entire body relaxes and there is a huge general improvement, similar to that produced by adjusting the head back to center on the atlas.

I can hear you saying, "If that is not quackery then what is? You will never make me believe such nonsense. Hocus pocus"! You will be surprised to find that in actual fact it is quite easy to prove that a crystal does in fact realign the bones of the skull. All you have to do is get some finger cots or rubber gloves from the drug store and carefully place your index fingers of both hands on the molars on each side of a person's mouth. Then ask the person you are checking to close their teeth very, very slowly and gently and stop when their teeth begin to contact your fingers on either side. If you do this very carefully you will find that absolutely everyone's bite is uneven, often very uneven. They will begin to bite your finger on one side a lot sooner than on the other side.

When you have determined which way their bite has misaligned and which side is tighter, touch the person with the fingers of one hand so as to pick up their vibrations and point the crystal at all parts of your subject's head and face. When you have finished, recheck the bite and you will find that it is now always completely even. It is important to remember that the crystal will have no effect unless you touch the person with one hand. You have to pick up their energy and their vibrations. You can, of course, adjust the bones of your own head by simply pointing the crystal at the different bones. It may be hard to do the back of the head. To do this you may have to ask a family member or a friend to do it for you. But do not forget that for the crystal to work, they have to hold the crystal in one hand and touch you with the other hand. If they do not touch you nothing will happen.

The skull is made up of a total of twenty-two bones. It is, therefore, important to point the crystal at all parts of the head. It is impossible to tell which of the twenty-two bones are misaligned and are causing trouble. In many cases just about all the bones of the skull are misaligned. If you point the crystal at all parts of the head, all the misaligned bones somehow, mysteriously, realign themselves. We will probably never understand how this happens but it is very easy to show that it does happen and also the huge, immediate changes for the better prove that in fact all the bones of the skull do realign themselves when the crystal is used as explained above.

Once again, by far the best and safest method of adjusting the atlas back to center under the head is called N.U.C.C.A method. All the other methods are terribly inaccurate and give very poor results or may even result in more problems. Therefore, you should find yourself a good NUCCA chiropractor. If you use your crystal regularly, to keep your skull adjusted, it will also be easier for the chiropractor to adjust your atlas back to center under your head. If you use your crystal regularly, you can make the adjustment hold a lot longer, with luck for years.

If you want to enjoy good health it is essential to have this done. The misalignment of the head on the atlas and the misalignments of the bones of the skull have an absolutely devastating effect on health. If not corrected they play an important role in causing all chronic conditions and they will gradually ruin your spine and your health.

The following two short case histories are good examples of the wonderful healing effects of crystals:

Case History #1 This patient writes: "I had chronic, constant jaw pain for over fifteen years. I visited several doctors but none of them could help me and they all said they could not understand what was causing my pain. When I began using a crystal my jaw immediately aligned itself and I have had no pain since".

Case History #2 "I have been treated without success by several dentists for TMJ problems. I could not hold my mouth open for more than a minute and going to a dentist was a nightmare. When I began using my crystal the pain stopped and my dentist could not believe it when I had no trouble holding my mouth open for the entire length of the treatment".

These two stories create the impression that only jaw

problems can be helped by using a crystal. The crystal aligns the entire skull, using it will help with all heath problems, to a greater or lesser degree.

SPINAL DECOMPRESSION

Because of the upright position we have to maintain, our spines become more and more compressed with time. This then results in pressure on the spinal nerves, which may in turn result in the malfunctioning of organs, weakness of muscles, pain, numbness or tingling of hands or legs and an endless list of other problems. Some of the typical symptoms are such things as shooting pains down the arms or legs, limitation of movement due to weakness of muscles, fatigue, headaches, chest pains, irregular heartbeats and more.

One patient wrote: "When I was forty eight I began experiencing a feeling of tingling in my left foot, numbness and extreme weakness of the thigh muscles. I could not raise my left leg. After many tests I was diagnosed as having inflammation of the spinal cord and I was given steroids to calm this inflammation. There was a marked improvement but when the steroids wore off the symptoms returned. I then spent thirteen days in the hospital having tests but the results were inconclusive. It was suggested that I may have MS but not for sure.

After about ten spinal decompression treatments most of the strength in my leg immediately returned and the tingling stopped. I have since spoken to many people who got very good results from different forms of spinal traction or decompression."

There are many different devices used for spinal decompression. Some large stores sell inversion units for less than two hundred dollars. Treatments on Spinal Decompressions Units in doctors' offices are probably the most effective way of decompressing the spine, but these treatments on very costly decompression units are also a lot more expensive.

You should do everything you can to prevent degenerative changes in your spine, hips and knees; they may not only affect your health but they may quite literally kill you before your time.

NOTE - It is important to use the crystal not only over the head but also over the entire body, arms, hands, legs and feet. If used this way the crystal has a wonderful balancing effect. When the crystal is used on the entire body there is an immediate improvement in the energy flow which results in a significant increase in the strength of many muscles. The crystal should be used more over areas where the skin has been damaged, e.g. scars, tattoos, stretch marks, calluses, piercings.

Remember to spend extra time on the area of the atlas vertebra. To do this, point the crystal at the part of your head just in front and just below your ear, on both sides. Always rotate the crystal in small clockwise circles. Hold the crystal about 3-6 inches from the surface of your skin.

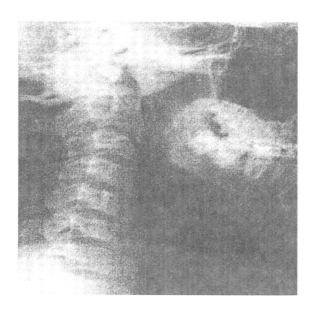

Illustration #1   This photo shows an x-ray of the cervical (neck) spine. The two main symptoms of weakness of the neck muscles can be clearly seen. A loss of the normal forward (lordotic) cervical curve and also irregularity. By irregularity we mean that the vertebrae are not well aligned and show a staggered or stair stepping effect. The line formed by the backs of the bodies of the vertebrae is called George's line. It forms the anterior or front wall of the neural canal through which the spinal cord passes. If the vertebrae are misaligned because of a weakness of the spinal muscles, as is the case in this illustration, there will be pressure on the spinal cord and the spinal nerves, with consequent interference with the normal flow of nerve impulses to some parts of the body. A neck like this is weak and the spinal joints are certain to wear out causing degenerative changes to begin at an early age.

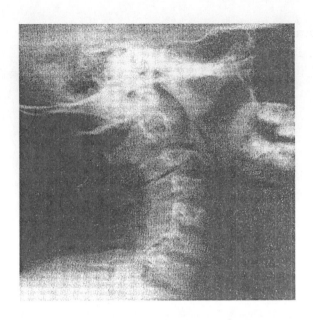

Illustration #2   This is the second X-ray taken of the same person three weeks later, after a program of daily exercises to strengthen the back muscles. It can be seen that once the back muscles became strong, they automatically pulled the vertebrae back to their normal, correct position and aligned the spine perfectly. The backs of the bodies of the vertebrae form a perfectly smooth line and there is no pressure on the spinal cord or the spinal nerves. As long as the back muscles remain strong and hold the vertebrae in perfect alignment, degenerative arthritis or osteo-arthritis is less likely to set in.

Notice the perfect forward curve. When the spine is curved this way the back muscles have so much more leverage that the back becomes, as estimated by engineers, twenty times stronger than it is when it is straight.

Everyone can have a good neck like this if only they form the habit of doing the back exercises daily. You should also go for a checkup once or twice a year to make sure that your atlas has not misaligned. School children should be taught the exercises at an early age. It is easy to develop a good spine while one is still young. The later one starts the more difficult it becomes.

The illustration on the next page shows the incredible effectiveness of back exercises. They have been taken from the book Ileopsoas by Dr. Arthur A. Michele M.D. and show a child with severe scoliosis before and after a program of exercises to stretch the psoas muscle and strengthen the muscles of the back.

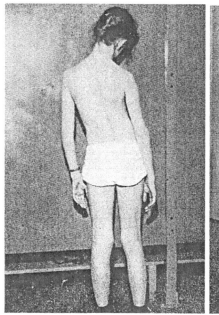 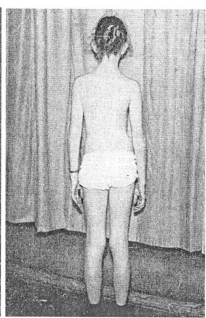

Before   After

CHAPTER 13
⌘
WHY BACK EXERCISES ARE SO IMPORTANT

It is essential to do back exercises every day. The back muscles have to be kept strong enough to hold the bones of the spine in place and in proper alignment.

If you do the back exercises regularly and make sure your skull and atlas is properly adjusted you will save yourself endless trouble and enjoy a lot better health. It is essential to form the habit of spending a few minutes in doing these exercises every day. If you do not make sure that your atlas is adjusted by going to a NUCCA chiropractor and you do not do the back exercises to keep your back muscles strong you will inevitably develop degenerative arthritis in your spine, knees and hips. This will not only affect your health but it will quite literally kill you years before your time.

To strengthen your back muscles lie on your back and then right and left sides and lift your head about fifty to a hundred times. Then lie face down and move your head up and down five hundred times or more. Use short, fairly rapid movements. Do not go all the way down and all the way up, that could cause you to become dizzy or even cause your neck to hurt. Unless you are a very fit person, you should start by doing only a small number of reps and then increase gradually, as you become stronger.

Weakness of the muscles which hold the bones of the spine in place is the main cause of so-called osteo-arthritis, or degenerative arthritis of the spine. This can be such a health destroying, debilitating condition that every possible effort should be made to prevent it.

Daily exercises to keep the back muscles strong are our

best way of preventing degenerative changes from taking place in the joints of our spine. As long as the back muscles are strong and they hold the vertebrae firmly in place it is impossible for this arthritis to gain a foothold. But once it is allowed to start and nothing is done to check it, it will spread like a cancer throughout the spine, destroying the discs and the spinal joints. Eventually degenerative changes in the spine can become so bad that normal function and health may become challenged.

Prevention of osteo-arthritis of the spine is one good reason why daily exercises to strengthen the back muscles are so important. Prevention of spinal misalignments is another. If the back muscles are strong they can easily prevent the bones which make up the spine and pelvis from misaligning and pressing on the nerves and spinal cord.

If the bones are held firmly in place because the muscles are too weak to stabilize them they will misalign and cause all kinds of trouble. This may not only just result in back pain but also in such things as malfunction of organs, headaches, numbness and a host of other problems.

SHOULD EVERYONE DO BACK EXERCISES?

Yes! Even if you are already very fit and already do a lot of exercise you should include the back exercises in your fitness program. In fact, athletes often have a greater need to do these exercises than persons who exercise little. This is because the main problem often is not so much weakness of the back muscles but uneven development of these muscles.

If the back muscles are weaker on one side than the other the stronger muscles will twist the spine in their direction. The spine can then become curved from side to side, this is known as scoliosis of the spine, the normal spinal curves are lost or they may become reversed. The back then becomes a lot weaker and more vulnerable to injury. Unless something is done to strengthen and balance the muscles, damage to the spinal joints and discs will follow automatically.

The main purpose of the exercises is not just to strengthen the back muscles but to strengthen them as evenly as possible. If this can be done the spine will be well balanced and it will never deteriorate.

When the back muscles are strong and well balanced your spine will automatically regain its normal curves and the vertebrae will be held firmly in their correct position. You will be surprised how much better you will feel. Your head will be clear, you will have more energy and your entire body will function better because there will be no interference with the nervous system. The flow of nerve impulses from your brain to all parts of your body will be restored to normal and it may be better than ever before in your life.

Amazingly, the back muscles are designed in such a marvelous way that when they are strong and well balanced the bones of the spine are held in exactly the correct position AT ALL TIMES; when you are standing, sitting, carrying a heavy weight, or twisting in any direction. This in itself shows that nature attaches a great importance to preventing pressure on any part of the nervous system which is the master control system.

Before starting any exercise program you should make certain that your skull and atlas are well aligned and are not causing your body to be misaligned. If you are misaligned exercises may tend to cause the muscular imbalance to become worse.

EXERCISES

The purpose of these exercises is to strengthen and stretch the spine and make it both strong and flexible. You should be careful not to overdo the exercises and increase the number of reps slowly.

When doing these exercises keep the following rules in mind:

1) Increase slowly as you feel yourself becoming stronger

2) Do not overdo. Only do that which you can do easily.

3) Only do short, fairly rapid movements. For instance, when you lie on your stomach do not lower your head as far down as you can and then lift it as high as you can. Just lower it and lift it, fairly quickly, well within your limits.

If you overdo you could get stiff, pull a muscle, strain ligaments, and become very sore. This could discourage you and stop you from continuing.

It is important to keep in mind that all exercises do not strengthen the back muscles. Frequently weight lifters and yoga teachers have the worst spines. To have a strong back you must do exercises which are designed specifically to strengthen the muscles of the back. Just being fit is not enough.

Exercise #1

Lie on side and lift head up and down 100 times. Avoid turning head. Remember short movements only.

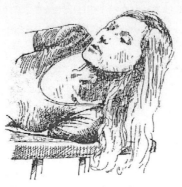

Exercise #2

Lie on back and lift head and body upper body 50 times or more up and down. Remember short movements only.

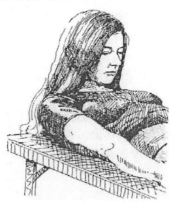

Exercise #3

Lie face down and lift head and upper body up and down 500 times. If you do this fairly rapidly it should not take more than five minutes. This is the most important of these exercises.

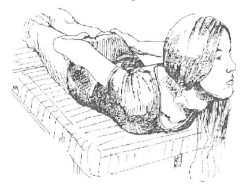

Exercise #4

Stand with your back to the wall and push back with your elbows. Keep feet about two feet from the wall. Repeat 100 times or more.

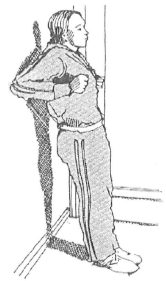

Exercise #5

Stand erect with arms outstretched. Rotate arms rapidly 200 times clockwise. Hold arms straight wrists flexed as far as possible.

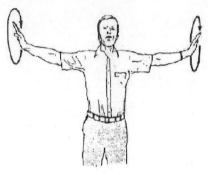

Exercise #6

Bicycle riding is one of the best exercises for lower the back.

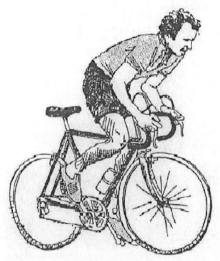

Exercise #7

Psoas stretch. Repeat as shown at least 10 times a day. Keep back leg straight and lean back as far as you can.

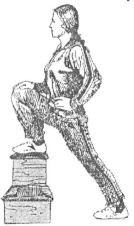

Exercise #8

Reach down to your toes at least 10 times a day. You can do this at any time. Be careful not to hurt yourself. Do this slowly.

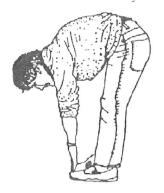

CHAPTER 14
⌘
AMALGAM – A POISON IN YOUR MOUTH

Many European researchers now believe that the highly toxic materials used in dentistry are an important, if not the most important, reason for the cancer epidemic of modern times. This is largely because there are many well documented cases of terminal cancer patients who recovered only when the toxic materials, mainly amalgam and nickel, were removed from their teeth. Before that, all therapies which were used on these people failed.

The amalgam scare has been gaining momentum for some time. This is because silver (amalgam) fillings contain fifty percent mercury, one of the most toxic and poisonous metals. Silver fillings were thought to be safe in the past mainly because very few patients showed an immediate allergic reaction to amalgam. If a person started having symptoms later, the relationship of the disorder to the silver fillings was hard to prove. There were no tests sensitive enough to detect the effects amalgam fillings have on the body. Since amalgam is very durable and easy to handle, it was conveniently assumed that it was safe. For some unknown reason, most dentists stubbornly insisted that all evidence unfavorable to amalgam was unscientific and inconclusive. The few dentists who tried to warn their patients of the dangers of amalgam toxicity were even threatened with the loss of their licenses.

Since electro-diagnosis and muscle-testing have made diagnosis more accurate, it has been possible to prove clearly the hazards presented by silver fillings.

These new methods of diagnosis have shown that:

1. Everyone, with no exception, shows a strong sensitivity to amalgam.
2. Even the smallest quantities of amalgam can cause serious interference with the energy flow in the body.
3. Amalgam fillings can cause abnormal changes in the body's electromagnetic field.
4. When the amalgam is removed from the teeth, traces of mercury can still be found in the brain, kidneys, and other tissues. ALWAYS!
5. The tissues close to the amalgam fillings remain chronically inflamed, all the time, from the moment of insertion.

Another important effect amalgam has is that it can seriously depress the immune system. For instance, in an article entitled, "Amalgam Toxicity: Grand Deception," Dr. Victor Penzer D.D.S. writes:

> In the pilot research by Eggleston, as reported in the *Journal of Prosthetic Dentistry*, two patients with depressed lymphocytes, had amalgams replaced with temporary fillings, and the T-lymphocyte count went up. When the amalgams were experimentally reinserted the T-lymphocytes dropped again. They improved once more when the amalgams were eliminated.

T-lymphocytes are white blood cells whose function is to fight infection and remove toxic elements from the tissues. The number of T-lymphocytes in the blood reflects the body's ability to fight invasion. From the above experiment it can be seen that amalgam can immediately depress the immune system.

The damaging effects of amalgams are often largely due to the interference they cause with the flow of energy along the meridian system. Therefore, the symptoms a person develops depend on which part of this system is affected most. In Germany, Doctors Voll and Thompson have mapped the relationship of each tooth to certain organs, muscles, and joints. They have found that if an amalgam filling or some other toxic material is placed in a tooth, a specific area of the body will be affected. This happens because the toxic fillings interfere with the energy flow to that part of the body, and results in immediate malfunction.

We have become so accustomed to accepting a second class state of health as the norm, that sickness has become an accepted part of lives for many people. If you ask these people whether they ever have headaches, indigestion, insomnia, depression, fatigue, irritability, backaches, or other aches and pains, they will look at you in surprise and say something like, "No more than usual! I am really lucky I enjoy good health!" It never crossed their minds that such symptoms could be caused by the toxic materials their dentist placed in their teeth.

I have spoken to a great many people who had their amalgams replaced with non-toxic materials. Most of them reported significant improvements in health. The symptoms which cleared up, after the amalgams and other toxic materials were removed from the teeth of these individuals, included: cancer, headaches, joint pains, backaches, fatigue, indigestion, menstrual cramps, hair loss, inability to concentrate, fits of rage, hemorrhoids, bad breath, arthritic pain, weakness, trembling, paralysis, enlarged lymph nodes in the neck and migraines. Dr. Max Garten, the author of several books on health, even told me that two of his patients who had been diagnosed as having multiple sclerosis recovered and were able to get out of their wheelchairs when their amalgams were removed. Leading homeopaths in Germany, who use electro-diagnosis, believe that close to ninety percent of the time, multiple sclerosis is caused by toxic materials placed in patients' teeth by dentists.

Recently candidacies, a yeast overgrowth, has attracted a great deal of attention. This condition has also been linked to amalgam fillings. There appears to be a connection between the presence of amalgam in the teeth and the body's ability to resist the yeast, Candida Albicans. When the immune system is weakened, Candida can multiply until it produces disease-like symptoms-such as aching joints, swelling, bloating, fatigue, headaches, etc. Removal of the amalgam fillings often produces a marked improvement in the symptoms caused by Candida.

Amalgam is by no means the only toxic material dentists use on unsuspecting patients. There are many others. The most dangerous of these is probably nickel. In a lecture at the Holistic Dental Convention, Dr. David Eggleston had this to say about nickel:

> Nickel is used routinely by national cancer centers to induce cancer in laboratory animals to study cancer. The nickel alloys they are using are very similar to those we are using in patients' mouths. Dentists are causing a major health problem.

Dr. Harold Kristal, D.D.S., whose practice is in Point Richmond near San Francisco, has done some of the most outstanding work on the problem of amalgam toxicity. In a talk on this subject Dr. Kristal said:

> "There are five ways in which mercury, from amalgam restorations, spreads throughout the body. (1) About 76 percent of all vapors that exude from the mercury fillings upon chewing are inhaled into the

lungs. (2) Particles of silver fillings that break off when we chew are swallowed and pass into the digestive tract. (3) If a silver filling happens to be close to the gum line, the mercury seeps directly into the arteries and veins. It then spreads throughout the body. (4) The mercury is absorbed through the dental tubules into the pulp arteriovenous system. It then spreads throughout the body. (5) The fifth and last way that mercury is transmitted to different parts of the body is through the nervous system. The vapors are absorbed into the Trigeminal and Olfactory nerves and pass along these nerves to the brain. This is very frightening because the simple vaporization from mercury can create various problems with brain function.

This work was brought up by Dr. Patrick Stortebecker, M.D., Ph.D., a researcher in Sweden. His book is called Mercury Poisoning from Dental Amalgams-A Hazard to the Human Brain. Dr. Stortebecker's work is very outstanding. He feels that many of the problems that we are having in our culture today are primarily brought about by the 150 years of mercury poisoning that has been thrust upon the human race. If you add this to the complex pollution that exists in the atmosphere today, together with other pollutants, you can begin to see the enormity of the problem.

It is felt that during the chewing process a person with an average of only three to five amalgams, may reach perhaps 10 to 100 times the toxic mercury levels that O.S.H.A. approves in ambient air in their various working places. Many people have as many as ten amalgams and in some cases many more.

I would now like to discuss nickel. Nickel is not nearly as active as mercury; however, it corrodes and is far more carcinogenic. The corrosion of those non-precious metals into the gum tissues, and then into the blood, creates tremendous havoc for millions of people.

One of the most severe known reactions to nickel toxicity is described by Dr. Eggleston. A patient presented herself to the Long Beach Memorial Hospital with kidney disease. She was diagnosed as having idiopathic glomerulo-nephritis. They called it idiopathic because they did not know what the cause of the kidney ailment was really. After examining the patient, her family physician suggested that she be checked with electro-diagnosis. When this was done it was found that she was highly reactive to nickel. The doctor asked her if she has any dental work done within the past seven years. She said that she has three porcelain crowns put in by her dentist. The doctor explained that porcelain crowns have metal jackets (made of a nickel alloy) underneath the porcelain and suggested that she have these crowns removed immediately. After the removal of the three crowns the patient lost all symptoms of kidney failure. This was one case in a million which primarily due to the nickel toxicity. This was poisoning her system.

I would now like to relate another case that I had myself. This patient had cancer surgery and had her breast removed in 1977. She came to me in late 1978 and I removed all her amalgam fillings. The only remaining restorations were seven nickel crowns in the front portion of her upper mouth. In 1984, when it became clear that nickel is a causative agent in cancer, I suggested to her that we should remove these seven crowns. However, before this was done a very exacting immunological checkup was performed. Six months after all seven crowns were removed, I did another immunological testing on her. To my great surprise I found that her complete immune system had strengthened amazingly. She had twice as many T-cells, twice the number of T-8 cells, and a much better balance of T-4 and T-8 cells. Her B cells also increased. In general, it is felt that if she had those nickel crowns removed earlier she might have had the immune system to fight and ward off the cancer.

I would like to describe another case that I had. A patient of mine, aged 65, was suffering from rheumatoid arthritis. She had a lower partial which was made primarily of nickel and cobalt. She had one tiny mercury filling in her lower teeth. This patient had only six lower teeth left, the rest were dentures. Full upper denture and this lower partial which was made of nickel and cobalt. I immediately removed the small mercury filling she had and changed her partial to a gold partial. Shortly after this was done she no longer had to take pain medication. She was on nine Tylenols a day. Even the mobility in her joints improved somewhat. This patient said that she traces the beginning of her rheumatoid arthritis to the insertion of that partial twenty-five years earlier.

I would like to describe one last patient of mine who has been with me since he was a little boy. Four years ago he came to me complaining of severe back pains and cramping in his legs, which made it impossible for him to do any physical work. He ran a large company and his restrictions presented a major problem. He said that he was going to many rheumatologists. They thought he had some kind of arthritis, but they did not know which kind. To be able to function he had to take strong pain killers during the day. If he did not he was unable to get out of bed and he could not get any work done.

I checked his teeth with electro-diagnosis and found him to be very sensitive to both mercury and nickel. I had used both of these materials in his mouth about ten or fifteen years earlier. Upon finding this suggested that we remove all these restorations and replace them with gold and composites. We did this and two weeks later he lost all pain. I can hardly wait for the day when these materials are banned in this country."

Toxic materials, such as mercury or nickel, play an important part in disrupting normal function. By checking materials-metals, acrylics, cements, porcelains, etc.-with electro-diagnosis, it is now possible to determine which of them cause allergic reactions and which do not. You should make certain that all materials used by your dentist are carefully checked before they are permanently installed in your teeth. Only amalgam and nickel have been mentioned here since they are by far the most toxic and dangerous materials used by dentists. However, some persons have been found to exhibit a strong sensitivity to many of the other materials used in dental restorations. You should make certain that your dentist checks everything he puts in your teeth with electro-diagnosis-gold, platinum, porcelain, cements, acrylics, composites, etc. Nothing should be permanently inserted in your teeth without first being carefully checked. For instance, you cannot "assume" that gold is O.K. it may not be. A leading homeopath once told me the story of a medical doctor who became violently ill and developed seizures because he was sensitive to the gold crowns in his mouth.

In his book, Naked Empress-Or The Great Medical Fraud, Hans Ruesch explains that because of the frequency of drug reactions and other complications which can result from medical treatments, modern medicine has become a leading cause of health complications in civilized countries. There may be some truth in that statement, but Hans Ruesch has overlooked dentists. Dentists cause infinitely more trouble. The toxic materials used in dentistry have a chronic debilitating effect on health. They act like road blocks on the body's energy pathways and make normal energy flow an impossibility. Everyone who has toxic materials in his mouth has to have health problems of one kind or another. They just don't realize it. Most people have become so accustomed to "normal headaches" and "normal fatigue" and "normal complaints" of different kinds, that they no longer know whether they are sick or not. They have never been truly well so they cannot compare their present state of health to anything tangible.

AMALAGAM AND THE THYROID

Since muscle-testing has begun to be used an unusual discovery has been made concerning the apparent effects of amalgam fillings on the thyroid gland. Muscle-testing has shown that even the smallest traces of mercury in the body seem to cause the thyroid weakness.

Muscle-testing is perhaps most useful when nutritional deficiencies have to be detected. By using this method it is possible to not only discover which deficiencies of vitamins and minerals a person has, but also precisely how much of each nutritional supplement should be taken.

When muscle-testing is used to check for supplements made of animal thyroid, most people show some need for this form of nutritional help. However, there is a great difference between those persons who have amalgam fillings or even the slightest traces of mercury in their body, and persons who are found to have no mercury contamination whatsoever. Those who have no mercury usually only show a very slight need for animal thyroid tablets. They may need just one or two tablets at the most, which presumably means that their thyroid is strong and needs little help. But persons who have amalgam fillings react differently. They always show a need for a very large amount of thyroid, often more than thirty or even forty tablets. But when all the amalgam is taken out their teeth and all the mercury is removed from their tissues (this can be accomplished with homeopathic remedies or with a soft laser), their need for thyroid supplementation immediately drops drastically, usually to only one or two tablets.

For some time, certain researchers have believed that hypothyroidism (a thyroid weakness) plays and important part in causing cancer. For example, in a lecture given to the International Academy of Preventative Medicine in Texas, Samuel Scwartz, M.D., presented his work, "The Incidence of Cancer in Patients with Thyroid Dysfunction". He pointed out that in his observation ALL of his patients who were diagnosed as hypothyroid (with below normal thyroid function) and were untreated, eventually developed cancer, within eight to twenty years. On the other hand, ALL who were treated (i.e. given supplemental thyroid) and remained on the treatment program had NO incidence of cancer. Dr. Schwartz also stated that hyperthyroid (over active thyroid) patients seldom, if ever, develop cancer.

Could this mean that everyone who has silver amalgam fillings and consequent thyroid weakness has to develop cancer unless they happen to die of something else first?

NO METAL IS SAFE

In the past, if a person was not found to be allergic to metals or other substances-when electro-diagnosis or muscle-testing were used-it was assumed that the material tested was not harmful. However, recently two interesting discoveries have been made which have shown that this method of testing can be misleading. First, it has been found that if a small sample of a metal or other material appears to cause no allergic reaction, this does not mean that a larger amount is harmless. Second, it has been discovered that even if the metal some jewelry is made of causes no allergic reaction, pieces of jewelry can cause serious interference with the meridian energy flow. This applies especially to items of jewelry which surround a body part-i.e. rings, bracelets or necklaces. This is because if an acupuncture meridian is surrounded by a metal ring of any kind this always affects the energy flow. The degree of interference seems to depend on the size of the piece of jewelry. For instance, a small ring will usually cause less trouble than a heavy bracelet. This is why many leading holistic doctors recommend that their patients, especially the more seriously ill ones, stop wearing all jewelry-even if it is made of gold or other precious metals.

The following testimonials are good examples of the harmful effects that even precious metals can have if too large an amount is used.

1. "I suffered with pain in my right wrist and hand for over ten years. At times the pain was so acute that I could not use my hand at all. On several occasions I could not sign a check because I could not hold a pen in my hand firmly enough to write. Although I enjoyed playing tennis I had to give up the game because of the pain I experienced each time I tried to hit a ball. Over

the years I went to many doctors seeking help, but none of them could find a reason for my problem. Eventually, a holistic dentist, who used electro-diagnosis, said that the pain in my hand was caused by a dead tooth. He suggested that I have the tooth pulled because it was causing serious interference with the meridian energy flow. He assured me that if the tooth was removed the pain in my hand and wrist would subside. After listening to his explanation and watching him check me with the electro-diagnostic instrument, I agreed to have the tooth extracted. To my great surprise and relief soon after the tooth was gone the pain which I had for so long ceased. For five years I did not have a bridge made to fill the gap left by the missing tooth and I noticed that my teeth began to shift. My dentist told me that a bridge should be put in before the teeth shifted any more. For a week or so after the new bridge was installed I felt no ill effects and I was happy to be able to chew better again. My dentist had carefully checked all the materials the new bridge was made of with his electro-diagnosis instrument to make certain they caused no allergic reaction. You can imagine my surprise when about ten days after the bridge had been installed I noticed the old pain in my hand was back, worse than ever. At first I could not understand what had happened and I did not even suspect that the new bridge could be the cause. However, when the pain did not go away, but kept getting worse, I went back to my dentist. This time, when he checked the new bridge, to his surprise he found that I was strongly allergic to it. After checking further with the electro-diagnostic instrument my dentist removed the bridge and once again the pain in my hand stopped. Further testing led to the discovery that although I showed no sensitivity to small amounts of the gold the bridge was made of, I was strongly allergic to the large amount which had to be used for the bridge. This large metal object (the bridge) in my mouth was also presumably blocking off the energy flow to my right hand and causing severe pain."

2. "Two years ago, for no reason that I could think of I developed serious health problems. I became weak and depressed and began having daily migraines. I was also covered in sores and welts which caused me continual discomfort. This deterioration continued and I became bedridden. Several doctors examined me and I was sent for tests, but nobody was able to find the reason for my problems. Then suddenly it occurred to me that my problems could be caused by a bridge which had been inserted not long before my sickness started. It covered five teeth and I could not think of any other major change which had taken place recently. My sister who was now living with me, urged me to go to my dentist and have the new bridge checked with electro-diagnosis. The dentist was surprised when we contacted him and said that he had checked all the materials he used very carefully and had found that I was not sensitive to any of them. However, he agreed to check the bridge when he heard how sick I was. To the general amazement of both the dentist and all of us, I was now found to be strongly allergic to the large bridge. When this was removed my problems soon cleared up and within two weeks I was back to normal. Further testing showed that although I showed no sensitivity to small samples of the metal the bridge was made of, I was violently allergic to the whole bridge.

3. Presumably, my body could tolerate small amounts of the gold alloy but larger amounts had a very adverse effect."

NOTE: Gum disease is mainly caused by a lack of calcium, vitamin C, bioflavonoid, and rutin, and not just poor dental hygiene. Electro-diagnosis and muscle-testing have shown that persons with gum disease, weak, tender, inflamed, bleeding gums, pyorrhea, or loose teeth are always low on the above nutrients. If you take enough bone meal or dolomite, which are good sources of calcium, and a supplement containing vitamin C, bioflavonoid, and rutin, you can prevent periodontal (gum) disease. You should take about 4000 mgs of vitamin C and 500 mgs of rutin daily.

CAUTION: Occasionally people have a chronic deficiency of rutin, which is the most important deficiency in gum disease, because of a sensitivity to the materials which have been used in dental restorations-amalgam, nickel, gold, etc. In cases like this the nutritional supplements will have little effect.

CHAPTER 15

⌘

PANCREATIC ENZYMES, NICKEL AND CANCER

About thirty years ago, a dentist, Dr. William Kelly, was probably the first to suspect a relationship between cancer and pancreatic enzymes. When Dr. Kelly had terminal cancer and he was given only a month to live, it occurred to him that cancer could be caused by the pancreas not producing enough digestive enzymes.

Dr. Kelly had a hunch that, like diabetes, cancer could be caused by a malfunctioning pancreas. In the case of diabetes, the pancreas does not produce enough insulin; therefore doctors control blood sugar levels in diabetics by giving them insulin injections.

Dr. Kelly reasoned that if that is what happens in the case of diabetics then cancer could be caused by the pancreas not producing enough digestive enzymes. These enzymes have two functions. They help digest the food in the stomach and the small intestine and they are also carried by the blood to all parts of the body. Their function is to digest and remove wastes which accumulate in the tissues.

Dr. Kelly reasoned that perhaps if there are not enough enzymes these wastes accumulate and form tumors. Therefore, if a cancer patient could be given huge amounts of pancreatic enzymes in the form of tablets then the enzymes would perhaps digest and remove the tumors. It turned out that Dr, Kelly's hunch was correct and after thirty days of taking huge amounts of pancreatic enzymes every hour, instead of dying, as predicted, he was cancer free.

Working on this premise, Dr. Kelly began treating large numbers of cancer patients with huge doses of pancreatic digestive enzymes, often with excellent results. He did this in spite of the fact that he was only a dentist and not a medical doctor. Dr. Kelly's excellent results infuriated enemies so much that huge sums were spent on taking Dr. Kelly to court over and over. Finally they managed to have an injunction passed in a federal court which prohibited Dr. Kelly from treating patients with his methods.

Recently, it has been discovered that nickel weakens the pancreas profoundly and cuts down its production of enzymes enormously, possibly by as much as ninety percent or more. From this it seems reasonable to assume that the cancer causing properties of nickel could be mainly due to its weakening effect on the pancreas.

Nickel is an extremely toxic metal which is used by scientists to produce tumors in experimental animals. The tumors are studied in an attempt to try and find ways of killing the cancer cells.

Amazingly, absolutely nothing is ever done to warn people of the very harmful effects of nickel. Dentists use it freely in metal dental restorations: crowns, bridges, partials, etc. Gold frequently has some nickel added to it to make it stronger and more durable. A lot of jewelry is also made of alloys containing nickel. No wonder we are having a cancer epidemic which is totally out of control and more people are dying of the disease every day.

The large laser removes or neutralizes nickel so it loses its harmful properties. This is probably an important reason why the laser is so useful in helping the body fight cancer.

SUMMARY

You should go to a good holistic dentist and have him remove any crowns and other metal dental restorations which could be made of alloys containing nickel. By filling our teeth with nickel and mercury dentists have played a leading role in causing the cancer epidemic of modern times.

Some doctors have found that if all the nickel is removed in some cases even large tumors will disappear even if nothing else is done. If you want to prevent cancer, you should either not wear any metal or place any metal objects that you do wear under a laser to remove or neutralize the nickel they may contain.

CHAPTER 16
⌘
THE AMAZING HEALING EFFECTS OF MAGNETIC FIELDS

Thanks to using electro-diagnosis, in Europe alternative doctors have found that when a person lies on a mattress which has a magnetic pad under it, in just a few minutes the magnetic pad will draw a lot of the harmful metals out of the body.

It is not surprising, therefore, that statistics show that people who use these magnetic pads have a far lower incidence of cancer and many of the other health problems which are caused by metals. This is further proof that metals are the most important single cause of cancer, MS and Alzheimer's disease. They also play an important part in causing just about all other health problems.

Magnets and the earth's magnetic field have an important effect on our health. For instance, a study, conducted by Dr. Gumiel of Project Genesis of the World Health Organization showed that insects lived five times longer in a ten gauss magnetic field. Human tissue cells also lasted two and a half times longer in the same magnetic field. The increased longevity is probably due to the reduction in free radicals which are known to cause aging. A ten gauss magnetic field is twenty times stronger than our current geomagnetic field. The current amount of our geomagnetic field (the earth's magnetic field) is extremely low, measuring only 5 gauss. It is getting weaker all the time as the years pass.

Dr. Dean Bonlie, a magnetic researcher, found that mice will die if placed in a totally magnetically deprived cage. In an 80% magnetic field reduction area, the mice went into slow motion, barely moving and also eating voraciously to survive. This definitely indicates the importance of magnetism as an essential environmental element. In the light of the greatly reduced magnetic field currently present in nature, it is wise to supplement it by having a magnetic pad under your mattress during the important restoring hours of sleep.

A small epidemiological study of 925 subjects was done over a period of three and a half years. There was a 76% reduction of new incidence of cancer and an 87% reduction of heart disease. This study was not large enough to be published but it is definitely of interest and significance.

By far the best, strongest and correctly designed magnetic mattress underlays (pads) are those made by Magnetico Inc. of Calgary, Alberta, Canada. This company has been doing research and making the product for eighteen years. Their toll free telephone number is 1-800-265-1119.

A properly designed magnetic mattress underlay (pad) significantly enhances the effects of the earth's magnetic field on our bodies during the important hours of sleep. Research done by Dr. Dean Bonlie showed that the magnetic mattress underlay causes increased oxygen saturation in the blood, faster wound healing, a reduction of pain and inflammation, less post-exercise soreness and increased toxic metal excretion. If you are unaware of how harmful metals can be, note the following report by a research pathologist at the University of Wisconsin. He found that lead and mercury were deposited in the arterial walls behind EVERY coronary plaque! This was consistent in 120 subjects who died from heart attacks.

SUMMARY

- **Fact #1**: The current amount of our geomagnetic field is currently extremely low, measuring only 5 gauss.
- **Fact #2**: Magnetism is essential to life on our planet.
- **Fact #3**: A properly made magnetic underlay can be made to enhance the earth's magnetic field to our bodies during the important restoring hours of sleep.

Any magnetic product placed on top of the mattress directly next to the body will expose one to both the Negative (-) magnetic field (natural to the north hemisphere) and to the positive (+) magnetic field (natural to the southern hemisphere but unnatural to the body in the northern hemisphere). Therefore, if a magnetic product is placed on TOP of the mattress the body will be affected by both fields, which is not natural, as half of the field will be in the wrong direction. As a result of this, it will fatigue the vitality of the person(s) using it and it will lower their immunity levels.

Magnetico's product is the only magnetic underlay that correctly restores a purely negative (-) magnetic field by being positioned UNDER your mattress, thus lifting your body above the peaks of positive magnetic fields between each magnet. The magnetic underlay is made up of many separate magnets all pointing in the same direction. It is placed under the mattress with the north poles pointing upwards to eliminate the effect of the south poles.

CHAPTER 17

✤

THE CAUSES OF HEART TROUBLE

Basically speaking there is only one cause of heart trouble, a buildup of cholesterol plaque in the arteries. It is true that there are other causes but they only constitute a tiny minority. The cause of heart trouble in most people is a build-up of cholesterol plaque on the walls of the arteries. When this gets bad enough your blood pressure may go up and if you like you can start taking drugs to artificially keep it down. These drugs may somewhat reduce the chances of a heart attack or a stroke but they may also cause fatigue and other side effects.

Although it is true that the drugs may keep your blood pressure down but the buildup of cholesterol plaque on the walls of your arteries has to slowly become worse so that the day inevitably has to come when you will wake up one morning with awful chest pains or some other very unpleasant symptoms. You may also experience these nasty symptoms at some other time of day, for instance after a heavy meal. At that point you will be rushed to the hospital by ambulance and you may be told that heart surgery is the only solution to your problem.

ALTERNATIVE TREATMENTS

Since the buildup of cholesterol plaque in the arteries is the main and just about the only cause of heart trouble and high blood pressure in the majority of people with heart trouble, the question is, "What can we do to get rid of the cholesterol plaque in the arteries?" Even better, "What could we do to prevent the buildup of cholesterol plaque altogether, so it would never even start?"

There are two things that you can or have to do. First, you must stop doing those things that cause the cholesterol in your blood to stick to the walls of your arteries and, second, you have to try and remove the cholesterol plaque which is already in your arteries.

It is now a well established fact that the amount of cholesterol in your blood is of no importance. Therefore, the cholesterol lowering drugs which are so widely used are absolutely useless. They are a wonderful bonanza for the drug companies but they do nothing for us.

The cholesterol only begins to stick to the artery walls if they are scarred. If they are not scarred the cholesterol simply passes through, no matter how much or how little cholesterol you may have in your blood.

The artery walls become scarred chiefly by chemicals, processed fats and pasteurized and homogenized dairy products. Therefore, the first step in the prevention of heart trouble is to avoid processed foods and foods which are contaminated with chemicals. Especially harmful in this respect are processed dairy products. That also means no canned foods, no fast food, no packaged foods of any kind, no sugar, no chocolates and no gum.

Another source of dangerous chemicals is water. The chlorine in water is believed to be especially important in causing scarring of the artery walls. Therefore, you should drink water which has had the chemicals removed, that is purified water or distilled water. It is also not good to cook in tap water. You should buy a filter to remove the chemicals which are found in the water that you use in your house for bathing, showering and other purposes.

You should also learn more about diet and food combining. Your digestive system is constructed in such a way that it can only handle one kind of food at a time. Mixing carbohydrates and proteins at the same meal leads to all kinds of problems, hardening of the arteries being one of them. There are many good books on proper food combining. Health food stores carry these books.

Eating lots of raw, organic vegetables and fruits, whole grains and no dairy products (cheese, sour cream, cottage cheese, and yogurt), no beef, and no free oils will greatly reduce the risk of heart attack and strokes. You should try to buy organic, locally grown produce whenever possible. Locally grown produce has not been irradiated or sprayed with extra chemicals when it is transported across state lines, which is required by law in the U.S.

REMOVING THE CHOLESTEROL PLAQUE

Very useful instruments are now available for checking the degree of cholesterol plaque build-up in your arteries. Many of the doctors who use alternative methods have such an instrument. This procedure only takes a few minutes and it gives you a good idea of your systolic and diastolic blood pressure and your heart rate and the degree of elasticity of your large and small arteries. The elasticity of the arteries is reduced by the cholesterol plaque. The more cholesterol is present, the less elastic (or hardened) the arteries become and the worse the readings on the instrument.

If your readings are not good, there are a number of things that you can do yourself, without the help of any doctors, to try and free your arteries of the cholesterol plaque.

CHELATION

Chelation is the name given to the process of removing the cholesterol plaque from the artery walls with chelating agents, mostly herbs and EDTA. Some holistic doctors use the

- Pressure on these nerves due to a thinning of the spinal discs in the lower neck, osteo-arthritic degenerative changes.
- Pressure on the heart due to a hiatal hernia or by misaligned ribs.

If these conditions can be corrected, the heart will often begin to beat evenly again. When the misalignment of the head on the spine is corrected, the contracted muscles in the neck may relax and the irregular heartbeats may stop. Traction of the neck can also be very useful. The hiatal hernia can usually be corrected by gently pushing down on the stomach. The ribs can only misalign forward and down. They should be pushed upward and back.

ANGINA

Angina has always been believed to be caused by something being wrong with the heart. Recently it has been found that this is not always true. The angina pains often stop if:

- The misalignment of the head on the neck can be corrected
- The pressure on the heart due to a hiatal hernia can be removed
- If the neck can be tractioned gently every day by lying on your back with a rolled up towel under your neck. (See chapter on back exercises)

SUMMARY

If you want to prevent heart trouble and keep your arteries free of cholesterol plaque you have to exercise regularly. Unfit, flabby people have far more heart problems than people who stick to a well thought out exercise program.

Make certain that your body is aligned by going to a good NUCCA chiropractor, using a crystal to scan your head daily and by doing regular back exercises. If you do not do this you may damage the joints in your spine and this damage will play havoc with your health sooner or later. Stay away from processed foods, combine your foods well and take chelating supplements regularly. Read books on nutrition and herbs.

Herbal teas are wonderful and will also help clean out your arteries. Catnip tea is especially helpful in many cases.

You may consider going to an alternative health clinic where they will place you on a strict diet and exercise program. This is a much more positive and helpful thing to do than waiting until you absolutely have to have bypass surgery and the toxic drugs that inevitably follow the surgery.

CHAPTER 18

⌘

RADIATION HORMESIS
JAY GUTIERREZ

I knew radiation hormesis was for me when Jay Guiterrez said "brain tumors are a piece of cake". All the other cancer clinics had given me only a 25 to 50 percent chance of success at best. Jay was another ray of hope in my hour of despair. People laughed at me when I wore rocks on my head and drank low-dose radiation water. Laugh if you will but it worked. The rocks killed the fungus which was contributing to the cancer and weakening my immune system.

There is a great deal of evidence that funguses play a part in causing chronic conditions and cancer. Fungus, parasites, Candida and bacteria destroy the immune system. I have seen tremendous gains in my energy levels. I am able to focus my attention better and my short term memory has also improved. My pain level is a lot better and I never have to take pain medications any more. My mood seems to be more stable and it is easier for me to exercise. My greatest improvement has been in my stamina and decreased dizzy spells.

My routine includes wearing the caritinite necklace, ear plugs, "hot rocks" on my head (close to the tumors), drinking the water and sleeping on two pads (crushed rock) that all produce the low dose radiation,

Low dose radiation has been shown to enhance biological responses, to enhance the response of the immune system, enzymatic repair, physiological functions, the repair of cellular damage including removal and prevention of cancers and other diseases.

The stone puts out between .05 and .09 mRems/hr and

does three things: provides a very low level of radiation hormesis, it absorbs and it puts out a very small DC current. The stones are great on painful areas, tumors and lesions. The mud packs put out between 1.0 and 2.0 mRems/hr for straight radiation hormesis. This works best if you simply sleep on the mud packs.

The water stone "thorium" puts out between 1.0 and 10.0 mRems /hr. Just place the stone in a gallon jug of water and let it sit overnight. What happens is that the water absorbs the radiation and only puts out about 0.06 mRems/hr. When you drink this water it will go through your body and will only stay for about three hours. It does not have to be any certain water and it does not matter whether you keep it in the refrigerator or not.

Nighthawk minerals has hundreds of testimonials regarding miraculous loss of pain, better sleep, increased stamina, cure from recluse spider bites, Lyme disease, MS and many types of cancers. Hundreds of people have killed the fungus in their bodies, rebuilt their immune systems and had other miraculous cures.

Bathing with the green "Eliat" stone using magnesium chloride flakes can be very beneficial.

Jay has now opened a health spa/clinic in Colorado. I will probably go there someday. I look forward to meeting one of my favorite people. He is full of love, hope and a great person to call when you are down. Thanks Jay!

Contact Information:
www.nighthawkminerals.com

CHAPTER 19
⌘
JEWELRY/COLORS

Although this has already been mentioned several times, it is impossible to overstress the importance of the presence of nickel, and possibly other harmful metals in the alloys used in jewelry, glasses, rings, ear rings, dental restorations (bridges, crowns and partials), watches, zippers, buttons, coins, and many other items containing metals.

Nickel is incredibly carcinogenic. It is used in experimental animals to cause cancers. If you have any metal on your body which is made of an alloy containing nickel it may be impossible for you to get rid of your cancer, and even if you do not have any cancer now, you are certain to get it sooner or later.

The following stories will give you some idea of the incredible cancer causing effects of nickel. A man was diagnosed as having a large tumor, "the size of your fist", in his right lung. He was scheduled for surgery to remove the tumor, together with his lung. A holistic doctor advised him to remove all metal from his body "since it could contain nickel". He was also placed under the low level or soft laser to remove or neutralize harmful metals in his teeth and tissues. When the man went in for surgery two months later it was found that the tumor had mysteriously disappeared so the surgery had to be cancelled. The diagnosis "Spontaneous Remission". A woman was found to have a tumor the size of a golf ball in her breast. When she was put under the soft low level laser and removed all metal from her body the tumor shrank to half its size in a week and soon disappeared entirely. Another case of "Spontaneous Remission".

You should have any metal objects that you wear

placed under a laser to remove or neutralize harmful metals. Especially important in this case are under wires in bras. In Europe it is believed that these under wires are responsible for many cases of breast tumors in women.

ARE YOUR GLASSES NOTHING
BUT A HARMFUL CRUTCH?

If you read books like <u>Better Sight Without Glasses</u> by Dr. Bates you will be surprised to find that it is often quite easy to improve your sight to such a degree that you can either stop wearing glasses altogether or use them only occasionally. Glasses weaken the eyes and the metal frames cause interference with the energy flow in the body.

There are a billion Chinese and few wear glasses---a fact that the Chinese attribute to special eye-massage exercises based on acupuncture. Twice a day, in virtually every school in China and in many factories as well, the Chinese stop everything they are doing and go through four exercises which only take ten minutes. They are asked to close their eyes, while dreaming of far off places, and begin massaging key acupuncture points around the eye.

These simple exercises are believed to increase the flow of energy to the eyes, relax the eye muscles and help to maintain normal blood circulation to the eyes. Researchers have been amazed at how few Chinese wear glasses.

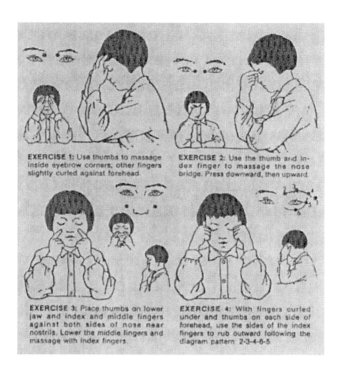

EXERCISE 1: Use thumbs to massage inside eyebrow corners; other fingers slightly curled against forehead.

EXERCISE 2: Use the thumb and index finger to massage the nose bridge. Press downward, then upward.

EXERCISE 3: Place thumbs on lower jaw and index and middle fingers against both sides of nose near nostrils. Lower the middle fingers and massage with index fingers.

EXERCISE 4: With fingers curled under and thumbs on each side of forehead, use the sides of the index fingers to rub outward following the diagram pattern 2-3-4-6-5.

When doing these exercises your eyes should be closed, fingernails should be cut short and your hands clean. Massage lightly and slowly and do not use excessive pressure. Repeat each exercise eight times, once in the morning and again in the evening, while sitting with your elbows resting on a table. You may find it more convenient to do these exercises in bed, a short time before getting up and again before going to sleep at night.

Most people have the mistaken idea that they need glasses because there is something wrong with their eyesight. This is seldom true, especially in younger persons. The real problem is a weakness of the focusing muscles and the muscles that turn the eyes in all directions. If you can strengthen these muscles sufficiently you will no longer need glasses.

Exercise 1 Hold your hand in front of your eyes with your arm outstretched. Focus on your hand and slowly bring it closer to your eyes. Then move it away again slowly. Repeat ten times several times a day.

Exercise 2 Hold your hand about one and a half feet away from your eyes and then move it up and down slowly while focusing on it and moving your eyes up and down also. Repeat several times a day. Then do the same while moving your hand from side to side. Repeat this several times a day also.

These exercises will strengthen your eye muscles and make glasses unnecessary. In older people the lens may become less translucent due to sediments or deposits. Therefore, the exercises may not work as well, so that glasses may be needed at times for reading fine print. Cleansing will help remove the deposits and improve vision. A person who went on a grape fast wrote, "After eating nothing but fresh ripe grapes for four weeks my sight and hearing improved so much that they were better than ever before".

NOTE - Anything made of metals interferes with the energy flow in the body, even if it has been treated with the laser. The laser will make it a lot less harmful but never altogether harmless. Take any metal objects off whenever you can.

The Q1000 hand held soft laser has a frequency for cataract removal and vision improvement. Check the laser manual for exact instructions. It reportedly has had very good patient testimonials.

COLORS

The Chinese were very much aware that bright colors can influence the energy flow in the body. Because of this, Chinese doctors are believed to have advised their patients not to wear brightly colored clothing for too long or too often.

It is now also known that wearing bright colors can cause deficiencies of vitamins and minerals. For instance, it can be easily demonstrated that wearing clothing of a certain shade of blue can cause a deficiency of iron and B vitamins, sometimes in as little as three or four hours. Red and yellow stimulate the thyroid and the adrenal glands and can cause deficiencies of trace minerals and B vitamins. The same could be true of other colors even if they are not so bright.

The conclusion appears to be that: if you want to remain healthy and well balanced you should wear mild colored clothing, at least most of the time. This will affect the energy flow in your body less and will help to keep your body in balance.

CHAPTER 20

⌘

FAR INFRARED HEAT

For centuries, physicians and scientists have understood that plants are dependent on sunlight to grow. It wasn't more than a century ago that Albert Einstein and other important scientists recognized the effects of sunlight on the Earth's atmosphere and human life itself. The sun's rays control vital processes for human health. The sun helps support the production of proteins, fats and sugars in our bodies. It stimulates the endocrine system, enzyme activities, various metabolic processes including the production of vitamin D.

Most physicians and naturopath's agree that the most beneficial and safest segment of the sun's energy spectrum is Far Infrared. The health and wellness benefits of Far Infrared are widely known and documented. Heating up your body with deep penetrating rays, Far Infrared waves (Bio Genetic) activate water molecules under your skin, vibrating through resonance resulting in vastly superior detox capabilities to safely help the skin detox many toxins and heavy metals through the sweat glands.

By heating up your body with deep penetrating Far Infrared heat, lymphatic flow and blood circulation are improved. This benefit alone enhances your immune system, increases metabolism, burns calories, reduces stress, encourages deep relaxation, improves sleep quality, and increases daytime energy and mental clarity.

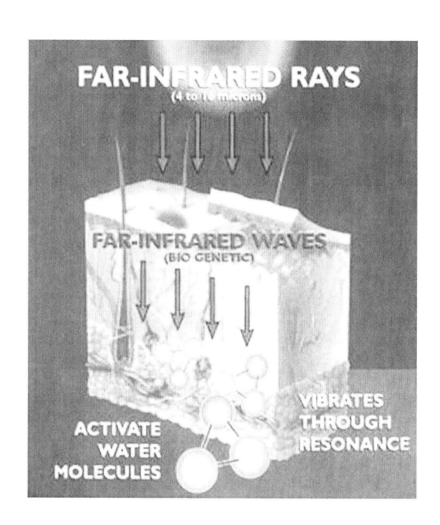

CHAPTER 21
⌘
CAREGIVER
By Sally Cole

When you are ill, one of the most important things in your life is who is going to help you. Having a major illness like cancer can be devastating to a person not only physically, emotionally and financially, but also in terms of your daily survival. Who is going to drive you to the doctors, clean your house, cook and grocery shop, take care of your bills and personal responsibilities and be your companion? Families are great but our children have their lives to live and families to take care of and cannot help you all the time. Many people are single, divorced or widowed and have no spouse to depend on.

A caregiver should be a person who can do all of the above plus be a friend you can cry and laugh with and complain to daily. Someone who will not judge you or become too close to be helpful. Having cancer or any life threatening illness is one of the scariest things a person will ever go through. No one should ever have to go through it alone. Find someone you trust with your life, because that is exactly what you will be doing. This person needs to understand what is involved in being a caregiver and how much time and patience will be needed. Major illnesses can last for years, not just months.

Being a caregiver is one of the hardest things a person can do. Caring for someone that you care about who is terminally ill and watching over what the disease puts them through is a nightmare. Trying to keep positive and jovial for them is at times heart wrenching.

The ability to be tough on them when they begin to go into a depression and feeling sorry for themselves and getting them through the hours when they want to give up and just lay down and die can be especially frustrating.

The caregiver has to be able to give so much time and effort. It is more than a full time job. It is a life changing event.

The caregiver must learn as much if not more about the disease and the treatments than the patient. The caregiver must come to terms with alternative medicine. It can sometimes look like "weird science".

CHAPTER 22
⌘
NEGATIVE EMOTIONS

It is a well established fact that memories of past misfortunes and traumatic events affect our health far more than most people can ever imagine. These negative emotions can quite literally make us sick even if we do everything that is recommended in this book.

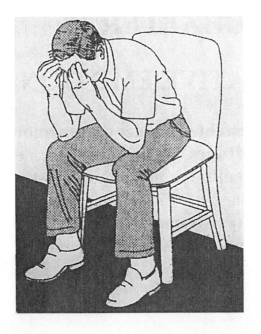

Eastern medicine recognized this and the Chinese found that the emotional points are located on the forehead, a little below the hairline on both sides. Eastern doctors believed that if one holds the tips of the fingers (all five fingers of each hand) on these points, as shown in the drawing, this helps remove or erase the bad effects of these past harmful emotions. When this is done they noticed that there was not only a significant improvement in health and the function of the organs but also a marked increase in strength of muscles. You should remain in this position for at least a minute or for a little longer. Doing this has a very beneficial effect on health. You should try and do it every morning and evening.

THE IMPORTANCE OF POSITIVE THINKING

Leading medical doctors believe that frequently our health problems are quite literally "in our minds" and can often be corrected by reprogramming the way we think. It is well known that positive emotions such as faith, love, forgiveness, acceptance, and happiness can influence our health immensely.

Every thought we think affects the function of the nervous system, the glands, the organs and the entire body. You will notice that the healthiest people are often those with pleasant dispositions whose focus is towards helping others achieve happiness and fulfillment, rather than selfish desire for personal gain.

Happy people do not usually give way to anger and pettiness. They use the power of their minds to maintain equilibrium. They do not harbor resentments over incidents of the past since their energy is being used to make the best of the present.

You could do everything recommended in this book, but if you continue to think in a negative manner, placing your attention on illness rather than on health, it could all be for nothing. Negative thinking can often literally destroy all the other positive actions you may take.

Health also depends on having worthwhile goals. If you can stay busy and excited about life you will remain healthier. When you no longer have anything to live for your body will sense this and it will stop functioning effectively.

Some people do not live long after they retire because they retire not only from their jobs but also from life itself. They fail to develop new interests and new goals.

Staying healthy and trying to improve yourself in every way is in itself a worthwhile goal. Few of us realize our full potential. We become depressed because of our lack of strength, endurance or mental power, not realizing that it is our duty to develop these talents. Disciplining yourself and giving careful attention to what you eat and exercise is not only beneficial for the body but also for the mind and spirit. You not only become healthier but also mentally and spiritually more fulfilled.

Your body has been amazingly created and it tries to adapt to every circumstance of life. If we work at it with courage and perseverance we can develop our god-given talents to an amazing degree. Helen Keller is one of the best examples of this. This heroic woman achieved impossible goals thanks to her incredible determination and tenacity. She did this mainly, or perhaps entirely, because forgetting herself she wished to help others.

Merely reading this brief comment on the importance of positive thinking is unlikely to produce a lasting effect on your attitude towards life and its problems. You should make a habit of reading books on developing positive attitudes and building spiritual strength. By far the best of these books is, of course, the Bible. In the Bible, God tells us of his love for us and his readiness to forgive all those who come to him and humbly ask him, no matter how serious their transgressions may be.

CHAPTER 23

⌘

THE BODY'S ONGOING BATTLE WITH INTERNAL AND EXTERNAL STRESS

Everyone wonders, "Why did I get sick, what did I do wrong?" The truth is that our entire life is responsible for our health. The bad things that happen can weaken us; they can destroy our immune system and open the door to disease.

I lived on Guam when I was 20 and picked up parasites that I carried with me until I was 60. I lived in Hawaii my junior year in college and got so sick from bleeding ulcers that I could not keep food down. I went from 130 to 105 pounds. While at California State University, Chico the next year I contracted Hepatitis B and had to be quarantined. A few years later my brother came down with spinal meningitis and I helped nurse him back to health. When I was tested at the Issel's clinic in Santa Barbara in 2008 my immune system was still battling Hepatitis B, parasites, mold, funguses and spinal meningitis viruses.

In 1978 my oldest son Matthew was born with collapsed lungs and he was on the verge of life and death his entire first year of life. I slept almost all that time at the hospital next to him. I also had the added pressure of my husband blaming me for Matthew's condition, even though the doctors assured him that I had nothing to do with it.

In 1980 I gave birth to triplets. I had a 20 month old, who was still suffering from birth problems, and now God gave me triplets. I laughed and cried when my mom told me that God never gives you more than you can handle. Well, I survived but my body suffered. The triplets were all full term and weighed in at 7-8 pounds each. The pressure from having them was so great that it displaced my internal organs, I still urinate quite often to this day, it broke one of the bones in my chest and I suffered with migraine headaches for many years.

In 1983 I divorced my husband after five years of verbal abuse: (on both sides) and took on the role of sole supporter for the whole family. My divorce was very high stress as the children loved their father. Divorce is a major immune stressor.

After marrying the love of my life in 1987, my husband Rich passed away in 1994. His death from stomach cancer was the most horrifying thing I had ever been through and aged me ten years. At times I still feel that I have not recovered.

Cancer can equal financial ruin for many of us. The next few years I went through a lawsuit with the medical insurance company for wrongful death of my husband. They had refused him medical treatment, when he came down with cancer, based on a drug omitted on the application filled out that same year. They called it "standard operating procedure".

I wrote the following letter to the court in 1995 while I was being sued by a hospital for some of my husband's medical bills. I was still a believer in allopathic (orthodox) medicine at the time.

SAN LUIS OBISPO COUNTY MUNICIPAL COURT
COUNTY GOVERNMENT CENTER
October 26, 1995

Your Honor:

As I watched Angela Landsbury (Murder She Wrote) coldly stare at another corpse of a friend hanging from a tree, I realized with much sadness how most

Americans have come to calmly accept the many atrocities they witness on television and around themselves every day.

Until tragedy strikes close to home, we are anesthetized enough to keep quite an emotional distance from it, probably an automatic physical response to keep us all from going insane.

I come before you, another member of the exponentially multiplying group of Middle Class Americans catapulted into poverty. We are dazed, confused victims of a decaying, sometimes corrupt system jumbled with obscure laws and contracts with confusing phrases written in print sometimes so small that most of us need a microscope to read it.

One beautiful Spring day in May, 1993, I quickly filled out one of those contracts. It was the first time I ever applied for my own healthcare insurance. It seemed simple enough at the time, a Blue Cross of California health insurance application. I was anxious to get my children's teeth checked. It had been almost a year since my husband had closed his failing business after 18 successful years, and I was repaying his years of support by paying for the policy myself. How could I have ever known that one piece of paper could so dramatically change the lives of my family.

MY HUSBAND IS DEAD. A good, hardworking man of Russian, Italian ancestry. I often thought that he secretly kept a book of Will Roger's quotes in his pocket. He loved America and he believed in her. He used to ask me, "Where else could a boy from the ghetto, Hunter's Point, San Francisco, grow up to own his own business?" He used to tell me how important it was for the Middle Class like us to support our government and pay some taxes. I quote "...because the rich won't and the poor can't... so it's up to us to keep the U.S. going."

Rich was my second husband. He was my hero and remains the love of my life. He died at 47 years old having raised his four younger brothers and sisters, two children of his own, and was doing a great job raising my triplets and older son from a previous marriage.

He should have died a hero's death. He served his country during the Vietnam War and served her equally well as a contributing member of the taxpaying community for over 35 years.

My husband's last words to me were, "I'm sorry", they should have been "I love you." He died believing that he left his family burdened with thousands of dollars in unpaid medical bills.

He died a broken man, not because of the cancer that consumed his body, but because of the loss of faith in the American system he so ardently supported his whole life. Rich never fully understood the circumstances surrounding that Blue Cross contract I filled out that cut off all medical treatment to him days before he was scheduled to take a pre-surgery test to determine what course of treatment would be most beneficial at that crucial point.

I died the day Blue cross refused to authorize payment for future and past medical treatment for Rich's cancer. Rich died several months later. He blamed himself, I blamed myself. After all, I was the one who failed to write down Wintensin on that form. A drug for the treatment of high blood pressure. I couldn't spell or pronounce it before that day. Now I can't forget it. Ironically, his heart remained true and strong until it pumped its last time on March 15, 1994.

Since my husband's death, I have been hounded by medical bill collectors, had my bank account attached by the state for my husband's taxes, have been paying $100/month to the IRS for deductions disallowed in past years that somehow came to light after his death, I made no attempt to dispute them, I have failed dramatically as a mother for my four teenagers, and my career as a real estate agent has practically become non-existent.

I consider myself to be healing and still only partially functional at this time. For over a year I sold almost all of our non-essential personal property. I spent the largest portion of this money on psychological and physical medical care for myself. I felt very suicidal, but knew that it would completely destroy my children if I did such a selfish act. I still believe when death comes it will be a sweet peace, forever ending **the memories that haunt me:**

--Rich's silence as he endured the constant pain…

--Pleading phone calls to doctor's nurses…only to be reminded of how much money I owed the doctors…

--The hatred I felt in my heart when my wealthy landlord insisted on putting our home up for sale while Rich lay dying, when I could not exercise the lease option, letting our $20,000 option money default to him.

--My angry phone calls to Blue Cross begging them for a written cancellation letter that never came so Rich could receive medical treatment at a County hospital.

--The pain and frustration on the face of the County hospital eligibility worker as she refused admittance to a man in obvious pain, his face and body swollen with new tumors as each passing week the cancellation letter never came. She was bound by a law that said no one with medical insurance can get treatment. If we cancelled the insurance ourselves, there was a waiting period before we could receive medical help...we needed that cancellation letter.

--Rich's incredible sense of humor. Upon his return from the dentist where the growing tumor in his jaw was probably mistaken for an abscessed tooth and Rich's teeth were pulled out, his smile as he consoled me by saying at least he got some pain pills.

--The long, frantic drive to the VA hospital in Palo Alto, only to be told that we made too much money in 1992 to receive treatment at that time. The counselor's systematic response telling us to come back in the month of January 1994, when our 1993 income would allow immediate treatment.

--The shock and confusion on my husband's face as one American failsafe system after another collapsed before us as a pile of red tape and little known, inflexible and uncaring rules and regulations kept slamming the doors to one hospital after another.

--The fear in my children's eyes every time we drove away, leaving them alone as we searched for care.

--Our second visit to the VA hospital in Palo Alto in January, 1994: the first time I ever saw a doctors eyes fill with tears. That shiny, hopeful face of a young female VA doctor as I helped my husband into the examining room. It was late; we had been waiting since early morning. She did the impossible-she got him an emergency appointment with the oncology department. She didn't know that much about cancer, but she recognized pain.

--My first complete emotional breakdown in front of Rich that same day, as the appointment clerk in oncology gave me a February date for Rich's emergency first visit with a VA oncologist.

--The saddened face of that brilliant young Stanford doctor at the VA hospital in February when he explained to us that it was too late for the expected surgery because the radiated esophageal area had formed a scar tissue he could not safely cut through. Consoling me, he told me that Rich probably would have died anyway.

--The JOY I felt as I held Rich's lifeless body..Peace had finally come...no one could hurt him anymore.

--The RAGE I felt on March 27, 1994, two weeks after Rich's death, when I opened a letter from Blue Cross addressed to Richard Gorkosky fully reinstating his medical benefits and apologizing for any Inconvenience the delay may have caused.

It is the perfect ending to this tragedy, to be sued by one of those hospitals. I have paid off many of Rich's medical bills at this time. I have on two separate occasions set up a payment plan with the collection company; but both times I was unable to make the payment. Ironically, the interest and added attorney fees are almost as much as the original debt. I feel confident that I can begin repaying the debt soon.

I would like to ask two questions. Are there any laws protecting the victims of this tragedy; and what steps can be taken to assure this situation will not happen to others? Are there time restrictions on healthcare providers for making critical decisions, as in the case of my late husband? Is there a way to press criminal charges? In this age of computers, I think that it should be criminal to take several months to decide on a cancer patient's suspension status. Please respond to these questions. Thank you.

I leave you with one final thought. As I watched The

<u>Rise and Fall of the Roman Empire</u> the other night, it brought to mind the comparison done a few years ago by a famous historian between the United States and the Roman Empire. I remember being impressed by the many similarities. The Roman Empire was far too powerful to be defeated by its enemies from without. It fell only when the people stopped believing in it-it weakened from its own internal corruption. We need to correct the problems within this country and give the Middle Class back its faith in America, for it is only with that faith that our country can be strong and survive.

Sincerely,
Susan Gorkosky

P.S. I have to take my hat off to President and Mrs. Clinton. Against the odds, they have at least dared to question the mighty medical monopoly that has this country on its knees. I pray that something beneficial for the Middle Class comes out of their efforts.

My first experience with cancer came in 1997 after three of the most stressful years of my life. They found a malignant tumor in my lung. Although the surgery to remove the tumor was successful it left me with a huge scar, about eight inches long, as well as feelings of sadness and depression.

High stress life went on with four children in college and houses to renovate and sell to make money. I was also experiencing a lot of back pain from the lobotomy so pharmaceutical drugs helped ease the pain.

In 2005 both my nephew Christopher, who was like a son, and my mother, who had lived with me for the past ten years, passed away: Christopher in an accident and my mother with Alzheimer's. That was a black year with tremendous sorrow and grief. My brain and bone cancers followed in 2007.

The United States started restricting our medical freedoms from its very beginnings which caused tremendous internal and external stress for us as individuals and as a nation. When our forefathers were writing the American Constitution's Bill of Rights the vote was tied on "Healthcare Freedom of Choice", sadly it was defeated by one vote. So the Constitution does not contain "Healthcare Freedom of Choice" as part of the Bill of Rights. Ironically two of the founding fathers died an excruciating death from the already ineffective and extremely toxic practice of packing the body with mercury to fight disease.

The American Medical Association (AMA) was founded as the union for medical doctors to fight for their existence as more people were going to alternative practitioners even then. The Federal Drug Administration (FDA) was set up to protect the people from harmful toxic/deadly food and drugs. How did these two separate entities become so entwined? When did we lose sight of the fact that the American Medical Association is just a union for doctors? Just like the teamsters union. It protects its own members first! It certainly is not synonymous with "truth, honesty and the American way". Yet it rules like a branch of our government. The AMA says it, so it must be the truth.

The FDA approved one trial for chemotherapy wafers that were surgically placed on brain tumors and touted as the next great brain cancer treatment. So I asked my doctor if I could participate in the trial and was told I was too old. They saved it for the younger, healthier patients. It had been put on the fast track FDA approval group of drugs for cancer. They all died, oops, another mistake! Thank God I was too old.

So many drugs, so many side effects. The number

three killer of people in the United States is hospital and doctor mistakes including pharmaceutical drug side effects, toxicity and drug interactions with each other that we still know so little about. We live in an FDA approved toxic soup. In the case of cancer, 33% of the people live longer who opt for no medical treatment whatsoever.

The pharmaceutical industry is a trillion dollar a year nightmare. The pharmaceutical companies fund doctor's continuing education classes, schools, government programs, and give incredible grants and scholarships to medical schools. Incidentally the average medical student has only one or maybe two courses in nutrition before he gains his license. That was probably why my brilliant MD Anderson trained brain surgeon told me to "go home and eat donuts," just enjoy my last weeks on earth. He really didn't know anything about nutrition or alternative treatments.

Pharmaceutical drugs try to mimic the healing power of real food and herbs. How can synthetic drugs compete with mother nature's healing plants, herbs, and foods? Why aren't we studying more about them than how to mass produce cheap synthetic imitations in laboratories and sell them for giant profits?

We are bankrupting our country with staggering healthcare costs. It needs to change very quickly. The system is caving in on itself.

I no longer believe in the current medical system. I use it for trauma (like my car accident) and testing since we are very good at these things. The rest of the healthcare system is broken. I still believe that it can be fixed. The human race is pretty good at survival. I hope we can survive the pharmaceutical dinosaurs that rule the earth now. Dr. Bruce Lipton author of Biology of Belief and The Wisdom of Our Cells describes these pharmaceutical companies so aptly as "small brains - big bodies". They can't even see that they are dying too with the bad water, bad food, and toxic drugs. We are all in this together. One of my favorite sayings seems to apply here, "there are no luggage racks on hursts." Even the Pharaohs of Egypt couldn't figure out how to take all their hoards of gold with them when they died, but they sure tried. Countless thousands of slaves died building those pyramids to Gods of Gold. The Gods of Gold are alive and doing quite well in our medical system.

Dinosaurs again rule the earth – insurance companies, medical monopolies, pharmaceutical conglomerates, oil cartels, all with their powerful lobbyists in Congress... who is in charge? When I asked for a single apology from Blue Cross the attorneys (I think there were seven present at my arbitration) told me there really was no single person in charge of anything. It was just policies and procedures handed down to them from someone "above" them. It certainly wasn't God. When the dinosaurs again become extinct perhaps this time we can include "Medical Freedom of Choice" in our new Bill of Rights.

SUMMARY

The events in our lives that can cripple our immune system can be physical, emotional or chemical (pain killers, alcohol, toxic foods, steroids, sleeping pills, most (or almost all) pharmaceutical drugs).

How we deal with grief, stress and anger can devastate our bodies and set us up for years of needless suffering and chronic diseases. In my case cancer of the skin, lung and then the brain and bone.

You must try to find some safe nurturing places and people, or just call a friend on the phone. Aerobic exercise, yoga, walking, swimming all help increase the joy in our lives. Chemicals released in our brains during exercise bring us some tranquility and rest for our minds as well as tremendous healing in our bodies. Do some mental housekeeping to rid your mind of all that past garbage. Prayer and meditation or perhaps a good therapist helps so much. I wish someone had told me that I didn't have to toughen up and handle everything alone. Chronic diseases start chipping away at our bodies long before the symptoms take us to the doctor.

We hopefully can include safe, non-toxic, alternative treatments in our insurance coverage so that everyone can afford to receive these wonderful treatments. Think of the lives that could be saved, not to mention the trillions saved in healthcare costs. More people now go to alternative practitioners than orthodox medical doctors once again. Preventive treatments should be covered through an insurance program. The current insurance companies cover few alternative treatments and none of them are for cancer. Why is that? We need to start another insurance company for alternative treatments. It could work.

CHAPTER 24

⌘

CUT BURN POISON
VS
NUTRITION THERAPY

"The treatments of cancer and degenerative disease is a national scandal. The sooner you learn this the better off you will be." Allen Greenberg, M.D.

Ever since I can remember we have been fighting the "war on cancer." Billions of dollars have been raised to find the cure. Yet, cancer is now the second leading cause of death in the United States and many other countries. I believe it's one out of three people will be diagnosed with some form of cancer in their lifetime. Most of them will die from it or the side effects of the current treatment protocols. Survival rates are dismal. The medical community keeps "dressing up the treatments" with fancy new names but it still boils down to radiation, chemotherapy, and surgery. These seem to be the only tools in their toolboxes. Orthodox medical doctors are literally locked into these treatments. Physicians can lose their licenses to practice medicine and be sentenced to prison terms for using other treatments. The following are excerpts taken from the DVD Healing Cancer Naturally from Inside Out narrated by Mike Anderson. If you do only one thing before making the most important decision of your life watch the DVD: Healing Cancer From Inside Out. It's an incredible two hours of information on treatment – conventional and alternative. I will attempt to synthesize it here.

"A cure for cancer is just around the corner!" Slogan from the early fifties cancer fund raisers.

"We look forward to something like a penicillin for cancer within the next decade." Sloan Kettering Cancer Center, 1953.

"There is a scent of victory in the air." Readers Digest article on Chemotherapy, 1957.

"We are so close to a cure for cancer. We lack only the will and the kind of money… that went into putting a man on the moon." American Cancer Society full page ad in the New York Times, 1969.

"… with a billion dollars for 10 years we could lick cancer." MD Anderson Hospital and Tumor Institute testimony to Congress, 1969.

"Cancer deaths can be cut in half by the year 2000." Peter Greenwald, M.D. National Cancer Institute, 1989.

"We are going to lick cancer by 2015." Congressman Benjamin Cardin, 2006.

"The medical community has been working on a cure for well over one hundred years. The war on cancer was simply a massive infusion of funds which ended up creating a bloated and massive medical bureaucracy…" Mike Anderson, 2008.

"The American public is being sold a nasty bill of goods. This is a bunch of sh--." Dr. James Watson, Nobel Prize Winner, stated while serving on the National Cancer Advisory Board, 1975.

"Research showed that chemotherapy was somewhat effective in 2-3% of cancer patients, primarily in the rarest kinds of cancer Hodgkin's, lymphocytic leukemia, testicular cancer, and choriocarcinoma." John Cairns, 1985.

"Some 35 years of intense effort focused on improving treatment must be judged as a qualified failure." John C. Bailer, M.D. of the New England Journal of Medicine, 1986.

"For most of today's common solid cancers, the ones that cause 90% of the cancer deaths each year, chemotherapy has never proven to do any good at all." Ulrich Abel, M.D., University of Heidelberg, 1990.

"Overall death rates from common cancers remain stubbornly unchanged – or even higher – than when the war began." E. Marshal, M.D., Science, 1991.

"Evidence has steadily accrued that [cancer therapy] is essentially a failure." N.J. Temple, M.D., Journal of the Royal Society of Medicine, 1991.
"We have given it our best effort for decades: billions of dollars of support, the best scientific talent available. It hasn't paid off." John C. Bailer, M.D. Harvard University, 1997.

"… the percentage of Americans dying from cancer is about the same [now] as in 1970… and [even] in 1950… Long term survival barely budged since the 1970's." Forbes Magazine, 2004.

"Survival gains for the more common forms of cancers are measured in additional months of life not years…" Fortune Magazine, 2004.

"Surgery, radiation therapy and chemotherapy... seldom produce a cure." American Cancer Society – Cancer Facts and Figures, 2007.

"The contribution of Cytotoxic Chemotherapy to 5-year survival in adult malignancies" – study of every randomized U.S.A. controlled clinical trial from 1990 to 2004. The medical community reported a significant increase in the 5 year survival rate. Cancers: Bladder, kidney, melanoma, multiple myeloma, pancreas, prostate, soft tissue sarcoma, unknown primary site, and uterus: 5 year survival rate 00.00%. Stomach 00.7%, colon 01.0%, breast 01.4%, head and neck 01.9%, lung 02.0%, rectum 03.4%, brain 03.7%, esophagus 04.9%, ovary 08.9%, non-Hodgkin's lymphoma 10.5%, cervix 12.0%, testis 37.7%, Hodgkin's disease 40.3% (clinical oncology, 2004 – absolute numbers)
*Note: Testicular and Hodgkin's represent only 2% of all cancers".

Generally the medical community thinks of a drug with less than 30% effectiveness to be no better than a placebo. Most chemotherapy drugs are far less effective than a sugar pill (unless we are talking about cancer). Chemotherapy drugs are touted successful with marketing campaigns designed to manipulate the "Absolute Numbers" so effectively that the average uniformed citizen believes we are winning the "war on cancer."

The medical doctors attack the tumors with a vengeance. The medical community has a "tumor fetish": shrink the tumor, cut it out or amputate the body part. Something is terribly wrong. The tumor is the tip of the iceberg. By removing a piece of the cancer (tumor) they must then try to get the cancer with chemotherapy and radiation.

By completely ignoring what caused the tumor "the medical community is leaving the fox in the hen house", Mike

Anderson, 2008. It will strike again. We all get cancer cells in our bodies every single day of our lives. Cancer cells are circulating throughout your body every moment. Our immune system is the only thing capable of destroying these cancer cells. A single cancer cell left undetected by a weakened immune system will start multiplying with astounding speed. Cancer cells eight year growth progression:

90 days – 2 cells
1 year – 16 cells
2 years – 256 cells
3 years – 4,096 cells
4 years – 65,536 cells
5 years – 1,048,576 cells
6 years – 16,777,216 cells
7 years – 268,435,486 cells
8 years – 4,294,967,296 cells

Most breast cancer is not detected by mammography until 4-10 billion cancer cells already exist. Mammography and similar tests could be called late detection. On the average a tumor detected is ten years old and has spread to other parts of the body (Journal of Surgical Oncology, 1997).

The first thing the hospital staff does is try to frighten cancer patients into immediate treatment, although the tumor is usually not life threatening.

"[Cancer] is a slow growing disease and they have time to think about this. The doctors put the patient in the position of thinking they have to make the decision in a matter of hours..." John A. McDougall, M.D., Dr. McDougall's Health and Medical Center.

Chemotherapy drugs are like flooding the body with pesticides. These drugs are so toxic that they are treated by hospitals as biohazards. Some cancer cells become very resistant. So new cancers appear later, the cycle of radiation, surgery, and chemotherapy are used again and again sometimes buying the patient a few years, sometimes not. 90% recurrence rates are documented. The FDA has deemed these drugs safe and effective for the treatment of cancer. A common side effect is death. "Bottled Death," Vice President Hubert Humphrey describing chemotherapy while dying of bladder cancer.

"Remember there are worse things than death. One of them is chemotherapy." Charles Huggins, M.D., Nobel Prize Winner.

Today it has become standard operating procedure to use treatments that don't work. These are the percentages of all cancer patients that undergo these treatments:

60% Radiation

67% Surgery

80% Chemotherapy

They have been pressured into using these procedures because they are the only thing available to them. Doing nothing at all, although usually better, is too scary for most frightened people.

Big money is at stake here for the pharmaceutical companies, the medical industry and big businesses involved in medical supplies and equipment. They want to keep these treatments as the only game in town. So they manipulate the "Absolute Numbers" by using terms like "making gains" to keep the funds pouring into their swollen coffers. They say misleading things like "the survival rate of one form of cancer has increased..." Scientific American, June 1987. In case of cancer the "cure" rate is given in terms of 5 years. "If you die of cancer in the sixth year you are dead and cured at the same time." Mike Anderson, 2008.

Early detection helps raise the survival rates in some cases past the "cure" 5 year marker. Cancer is the only disease in the history of the world to be said to be cured if you can live with it for five years or longer.

"You can fool some of the people all of the time... and these are the ones you want to concentrate on." G.W. Bush

The use of "Relative Benefit" instead of "Absolute Numbers" is a deceptive marketing tool used to make a drug look like its working. In a clinical drug trial 100 people are given a drug to prevent some type of cancer. Two were expected to get cancer <u>or</u> 2%. When only one got cancer:

1 in 100   =1%

2 in 100   1÷2=50% Relative Benefit, so this is the 50% we always see advertised.

One such trial was that of a breast cancer drug called Tamoxifen. Headline articles came out about this new breakthrough drug for cancer prevention. After five years of taking Tamoxifen the (Relative Benefit) 49% decrease in breast cancer occurrences was announced: In fact, the Absolute Number benefit was 1.5%, less than a sugar pill. Side effects included liver and uterine cancer.

Ask your doctor for Absolute Numbers. Ask him how many months or days will these drugs buy you. Most doctors believe these Rubber Numbers fed to them by the pharmaceutical companies. It is hard for doctors to say they have nothing to offer the cancer patients. Everybody is doing well in the cancer business except the patients. American Cancer Society is the wealthiest nonprofit organization in the world.

The enforcement arm of the cancer industry is the Food and Drug Administration (FDA) their track record for approval of toxic cancer drugs is astounding. They shut down any promising natural cancer therapies like Laetrile or Vitamin C. Now all other natural cancer treatments are illegal and enforced by the FDA for the "corporate medicine will not allow a cure for cancer." Mike Anderson, 2008.

NUTRITION – CONTROLS EXPRESSION OF BAD GENES

Poor diet and lifestyle wake up bad genes. You can put them back to sleep by developing simple diet and lifestyle changes. If we continue to fertilize these bad genes, we will continue to get cancer and other degenerative diseases.

Historical Percent of Calories
　　　Animal Foods　　　　　　　5%
　　　Refined Foods　　　　　　　0%
　　　Whole Plant Based Foods　95%
Current Percent of Calories
　　　Animal Foods　　　　　　　42%
　　　Refined Foods　　　　　　　51%
　　　Whole Plant Based Foods　7%
　　　(Cancer and other degenerative diseases have skyrocketed)

Whole Plant Foods
Fiber
Antioxidants
Misc Cancer Fighters
Low Fat
Low Protein
Low Toxins
No Hormones

Animal/Refined Foods
No Fiber
No Antioxidants
No Cancer Fighters
High Fat
High Cholesterol
High Protein
High Toxins
High Hormones

Some people find it easy to believe that eating a plant based diet can prevent cancer. They don't, however, believe they can reverse cancer by changing their diet.

Diets were first seriously studied for heart disease to prove that heart disease could be reversed with a plant based diet. Dr. Coldwell Esselstyn took 12 of the worst coronary heart disease patients that modern medical institutions could throw at him and he cured 11 of them through diet. The 12th patient did not follow the planned diet and died. They followed a very strict plant based diet. The diet is outlined in his book, <u>Prevent and Reverse Heart Disease.</u> Dr. Dean Ornish's book <u>Program for Reversing Heart Disease</u> also discusses dietary changes. Yet although it has been proven adopting a plant based diet reverses heart disease, the medical industry still uses the expensive bypass surgeries, stents and statin drugs as its first line of defense for fighting the nations #1 Killer: Heart Disease. Big money rules as people are mere pawns in this corrupt system. People believe their doctors – doctors are trained by the pharmaceutical and medical industries.

Adult onset diabetes is another perfect example of the medical system at work. They will tell patients there is no cure for their Type II Diabetes. You must take drugs for life. What they should be saying is there is no drug that can cure it. Most doctors agree that the Standard American Diet (SAD) causes it. Doctors just fail to tell their patients to go to a plant based diet to cure it.

Weimar Institute, Hippocrates Health Institute, Gerson Institute and many others put their guests on a raw foods, plant based diet and will get them off their insulin drugs within a week.

Diet is the "Elephant" in the kitchen. The average person with a healthy immune system usually fights off serious cancers in their bodies several times without even knowing it.   A healthy organic, whole plant based diet can win major victories over most chronic diseases.   The foundation of a well-functioning immune system is diet.   It multiplies immune system cells which fight cancer every day of our lives.

In one study breast cancer patients were divided into two group's one group was asked to remain on the Standard American Diet (SAD) and the other half was asked to begin an all plant based diet.   After only 4 years 40% on the SAD had recurrences of breast cancer while the group who switched to the plant based diet had not a single recurrence of breast cancer. Similar statistics apply to studies done on melanoma, colon, pancreatic, and prostate cancers.

Animal protein is the strongest carcinogen known. Low rates of protein = low rates of cancer. T. Colin Campbell found through his research that not only could he prevent liver cancer in his clinical study with mice but by raising and lowering the levels of casein (cows milk) during his clinical trials he could turn cancer on or off like a light switch.   T. Colin Campbell's book, The China Study goes into amazing details and his research spans thousands of people and over thirty years of research. It is the largest nutritional study ever conducted. Research studies found that no matter how many carcinogens entered the body, the development of cancer was dependent on how much animal protein was consumed. Animal protein makes us more susceptible to cancers of every type, also heart disease, and other degenerative diseases escalated with the increase in animal protein consumption. Plant based diets protect us from cancer. Nutrients from plant foods shrink tumors, while nutrients from all animal foods grow tumors.

According to Dr. Campbell our reverence for animal protein seems to be behind most illnesses in the modern American culture. Animal protein increases the activity of the enzyme in our liver called <u>mixed function oxidase</u> which has the capability to turn off and on the cancer cells, impairs the immune system's Natural Killer Cells production (the "big gums" for fighting cancer), increases estrogen hormone levels, modulates energy levels. All combine to make the diet of primary importance to our health. Eating animal protein takes a lot of enzymes to digest it. It can cause a shortage of pancreatic enzymes in the body. Digesting animal protein requires the digestive enzymes trypsin and chymotrypsin.

Cancer cells hide in the body because of the protective protein coating around them. The pancreas produces two enzymes trypsin and chymotrypsin necessary to digest the protein coating around the cancer cells making the cancer cells then visible to the immune system so they can be destroyed. Digesting animal protein competes for the same enzymes that fight the cancer.

Pancreatic enzymes are not necessary to digest vegetable protein so you can eat as much as you want. If you want cancer to stay in remission, change your diet and lifestyle for good. An organic plant based diet with <u>no animal protein</u> will make sure those cancer cells protective protein coatings continue to be eaten by the pancreatic enzymes thereby exposing the cancer cells to the body's fantastically efficient immune system.

The cancer is only invisible when that protective protein shell remains intact. You need to keep those cancer cells exposed and vulnerable. The body's Natural Killer Cells will make sure those cancer cells are destroyed every day for the rest of your life.

Positive attitude is a key to successfully healing your body. The placebo effect can be a very powerful healer. Remember Norman Cousens healed himself of terminal cancer by laughing with the Marx Brothers. Depression doubles the risk of cancer.

Mind-Body-Spirit are all important pieces. Each piece needs to be balanced. Each piece plays its own vital role in keeping our immune system strong and ready to deal with those ever present cancer cells.

Make the change to a healthy plant based diet fun. Don't look at it as work, it's just new. Soon your taste buds will crave the goodness and vibrant taste of truly good food.

"Every cell in your body is eavesdropping on your thoughts." Depak Chopra, M.D.

CHAPTER 25

⌘

MY DAILY ROUTINE

"Healing from a chronic condition takes patience, work and complete focus every day." It is more than a full time job. I know this because I experimented with dozens of immune building protocols.

Some of them were okay but too labor intensive for me. I was just too sick to do some things. I am sure that I left some great treatments by the wayside. With cancer you are fighting the clock. You have to choose your game plan and then give it time to work. I chose mine by what my body could tolerate. Some things were eliminated because I felt so weak, or my brain felt as if it was going to explode. I put together my own daily routine of what worked for me. I trusted my "gut feelings" (right or wrong) when choosing the treatments for myself.

1. Imprinter on arising and after every meal
2. Dry brush skin and shower
3. Wheatgrass juice – 2oz morning and evening, (2oz in enema water, 4oz implant once per week)
4. Lemon water with 1Tbs ground flaxseed, stevia, cayenne pepper and probiotic
5. 16 oz glass rock water
6. HIXI (20 drops) Waiora Cellular Defense (10 drops)
7. Imprinter, hold under bowl or plate of food every meal
8. Fresh organic juices: lemon with stevia, cucumber, HHI recipe, green vegetable (kale, romaine lettuce, red cabbage, red bell peppers, sunflower sprouts,

pea shoots, cucumber, ginger, garlic cloves, turmeric root, daikon root, parsley, spinach, leafy greens)

9. Breakfast(juices)/Lunch/dinner 80% organic raw vegetables, sprouts, soaked and sprouted whole grains, nuts and seeds, sea vegetables, 20% steamed vegetables, cooked whole grains, brown rice, quinoa (organic if possible – less toxic, more nutritious), sprouted bean soups, fresh sprouted bread, occasional: organic fruit or ice cream (frozen bananas or nut milk)

10. Laser, Q1000, daily 1-2 hours over entire body; use both enhancers at least 9 minutes each: 808 for head and bones, 660 over entire body

11. Ionic foot bath 2-3 times a week

12. Far infrared sauna 2-3 times a week 128 degrees 60 minutes

13. Lymphatic massage once a week

14. Acupuncture once a week with Q1000 laser with 660 attachment

15. Rub scars daily with vitamin A&E or coconut oil.

16. Digestive enzymes 30 minutes before each meal

17. Systemic enzymes morning/evening on an empty stomach

18. Steam distilled water with trace minerals 8-10 glasses

19. Morning walk 3 miles every day. Yoga, swimming, strength training 5x per week for 1 hour

20. Whole food supplements as directed on bottles (only take what I need based on blood tests)

21. Juice fast on Wednesday – water and juices only

22. Daily meditation, prayer and positive affirmations

23. Listening to inspirational CDs, reading a great book (there are so many), or journaling

My favorite affirmation: "I am whole, perfect, healthy, strong, loving, harmonious, happy and grateful." I modified it from one that I heard on the CD "The Secret."

I do not watch news channels on television, instead I listen to lots of inspirational and 70's music and Eckhardt Tolle's books on CD for meditation when my mind won't settle down.

Buying your own entire houseful of these things is still less expensive than one month at Issel's Clinic. So if money is an issue you can skip the high cost of clinics and do the body work yourself or with a caregiver. The tools I mentioned: the Q1000 laser with attachments, the imprinter, the crystal, low dose radiation stones, sauna, ionic foot bath and enema kit will run you under 15,000 dollars. The Q1000 laser has an acupuncture attachment that stimulates the lymphatic system and bathes your body in healing, soft light energy. The far infrared sauna treatment costs 25-40 dollars per session. Some gyms now have them.

CHAPTER 26
✿
ADDITIONAL SUPPLEMENTATION

MAXAM NEUTRACEUTICALS
PCA

1. Removes heavy metals
2. Attaches to and removes many harmful toxins
3. Removes cardio and cerebral vascular plaque
4. Helps rid the body of harmful mycoplasmas
5. Lowers elevated enzyme counts
6. Helps those suffering from various environmental illnesses
7. Provides a less invasive form of chelation

PCA is Maxam Lab's breakthrough solution to toxicity in the body. Without knowing it, people go through life involuntarily collecting a variety of toxins, metals and other contaminants in their bodies. Everyday circumstances: like the air we breathe, the food we eat, diseases, vaccinations, prescription drugs and even the place each of us calls home, all contribute to the degree of toxic exposure we can experience and eventually suffer from. Some of the harmful contaminants that can silently accumulate in the body include: heavy metals (such as lead, mercury, aluminum) toxic chemicals, inoculation residues, plaque, pesticide remnants, and many others, all of which collect in our cells. PCA effectively, naturally, and gently removes all of these contaminants and any others that are not a natural part of our makeup.

The result of years of rigorous research and

development, PCA is a living bacterial organism in a bottle - a powerful yet safe alternative to traditional chelation therapy.

It utilizes the unique concept of clathration to cleanse the body of this unwanted and often dangerous toxicity. While chelation is usually achieved with drugs and chemicals, PCA is a living formula actually made up of helpful bacteria and other microbes that, when used, become a natural, living part of the body's immune system. PCA is the most effective nutritional support product available for physiological toxin removal and cleansing.

PCA has also been found to have a miraculously positive effect on the symptoms which result from environmental illnesses and other conditions where toxic exposure is suspected. (*Maxam Labs excerpt)

Just four sprays under the tongue in the morning and evening, what an incredibly easy way to achieve total detoxification.

PROBIOTICS

Probiotics is another great product from MAXAM Labs. Its live 5-year fermentation process combines micro-activated strains of lactic bacteria with 92 specifically chosen vegetables, fruits, seaweeds, leaves, barks, herbs and spring water harvested from the mountains and seas of Japan. It provides four organic acids (including lactic acid) to establish proper colon pH, 10 vitamins, 8 minerals, 18 amino acids, FOS and other essential probiotics. It is stronger than any other probiotic on the market today. It is a biologically active, fermented paste with the same nutritional potency as its original raw food state (no unhealthy drying process).

Probiotics are essential to re-colonize the intestinal probiotic flora necessary for proper digestion and proper utilization of nutrients. Pharmaceutical drugs, antibiotics and toxins from many sources deplete the body of necessary probiotics. They should be replenished daily.

Probiotics is rich with "raw-food" nutrition, vegan and doesn't need to be refrigerated (that way I remember to take it). Find out more about it at maxamlabs.com or call (800) 800-9119. Julie Graves is the general manager there and is a fountain of great information. Five years ago she had advanced breast cancer and used these products as part of her protocol to regain her health. She was so impressed with her results that she decided to join the Maxam Lab management team. Today, she works tirelessly to help people with all kinds of diseases. She's wonderful.

WAIORA
Natural Cellular Defense and H1X1

In my line of work, real estate and construction, I was exposed to every conceivable heavy metal and carcinogens like black mold, mildew, fungus and fumigation toxins on a daily basis. I rarely wore protective masks, like most construction workers, they were just too hot and bulky. I never gave a thought to the damage they could do to my body.

Natural Cellular Defense came to the rescue as an adjunct to the laser, the foot bath and the imprinter. When I added the NCD drops it made a big difference, I felt stronger and better every day.

I was introduced to NCD and the mushroom H1X1 by my girlfriend Shelley at the Integrative Wellness Center. The first time I took the mushroom, I felt an instant trickling down the back of my head and it scared me. At this point everything scared me. I called Shelley and she told me it was working and had gone straight to the tumors. Again, as with everything I am doing, it is a wonderful immune system rebuilder. I now take it every day and will do so for the rest of my life.

Zeolites are naturally occurring crystalline minerals commonly found in rock deposits; they are formed over millions of years by the crystallization of volcanic rock and ash as they come in contact with salt of fresh water.

Zeolite has been found to be capable of selectively attracting and binding toxic particles, whether they are heavy metals, radioactive particles viruses, or other carcinogens that may be contributing factors to chronic illness, and safely removing them before they can harm us. Not only does zeolite help eliminate toxic build-up, it has also been found to help control blood sugar levels, balance the body's ph, improve digestion and absorption, support healthy immune function, help allergies and improve the body's resistance to cancer.

Toxins come from a variety of sources even our air, food and water are polluted. Some of our top toxic threats are heavy metals, pesticides, herbicides, dioxides and furans.

Because chemicals and exposure to toxins are impossible to avoid the use of detoxifying and chelating agents such as activated, liquid zeolite should be a part of everyone's life. There is no better gift that you can give yourself and your loved ones.

Scientists have studied the health potential of medicinal mushrooms such as reishi, shitake and maitake mushrooms, but the most health-promoting mushroom, the Agaricus Blazei, comes from Brazil. It has superior nutritional and antioxidant value and it contains over one hundred key nutrients. Experts recommend taking Agaricus liquid over nutritional supplements as this form delivers more of the healing properties.

Agaricus Blazei H1X1 liquid can help with cholesterol control and help reduce the effects of chemotherapy and radiation. It is a great source of health-promoting beta-glucans, assists in detoxifying the body, protects against bacteria and viruses, possesses antioxidant potential, boosting the immune system and directly attacking cancer cells, particularly cancer-cell apoptosis and cytotoxicity.

ENZACTA
PXP

Enzacta's Alpha PXP Forte is a blend of polysaccharide peptides derived from selected rice grains from the Siam Valley of Thailand and Spirulina from the Pacific Ocean (one of David Wolfe's "super foods"). This powerful mixture combines over 50 antioxidants, second-generation amino acids and alpha glycans. PXP uses state-of-the-art nanotechnology to bond polysaccharide peptides, through a patented hydrolization technique, to form powerful, concentrated alpha glycans. Alpha glycans are tiny nutrients that are easily absorbed by your cells which recognize them as "super-fuel-nutrients". You just can't get this kind of nutrition absorption in the standard American diet (SAD).

This "super fuel" is pumped directly into the cellular mitochondria, the power plant of your cells, producing a flood of pure, healthy energy from the alpha glycans. Powerful protection is provided by over 50 antioxidants which neutralize free radicals (those dangerous toxins that rip through your cells and cellular DNA, causing cell damage, mutation and premature cell death). Free radicals are linked to degenerative diseases like cancer, heart disease, Alzheimer's, stroke, diabetes and many more.

Most of us, particularly those of us with chronic illnesses like cancer, are starving to death at the cellular level. Our digestive systems are so compromised that we are lucky to absorb 20% of the nutrients that we eat, this includes supplements, vitamins, and minerals. Juicing is so vital because we absorb about 85% of the nutrients. Unfortunately, juicing is difficult at times (traveling, too tired, no good fresh organic vegetables available.). Alpha PXP, because of nanotechnology, contains particles so small that they enter the cell with nutrient absorption at 99.9%.

PXP is an amazing food. It supports cellular function, repair and restoration. Proper cellular nourishment helps the body's ability to boost the immune system to fight disease, increase energy, vitality, mental clarity and focus. It also enhances brain functions, decreases high blood pressure, balances blood sugars, improves digestion, boosts metabolism, increases weight loss and slows aging the natural, healthy way (my fading red hair is getting red again).

This product is sold through a multilevel marketing organization. Many new, exceptionally good products are using this marketing method to reach as many people as possible in the shortest amount of time, with the greatest dissemination of information. If this product went on the shelf at a health food store, the true value would probably get lost in the myriad of "great or not so great" products. For more information email me at sgorkosky@att.net. Enzactausa.com has loads of great information.

SIMPLEXITY HEALTH: APHANIZOMENON FLOS-AQUAE

Simplexity Health is the premium source for one of the planet's most powerful superfoods. This ancient freshwater botanical is harvested in only a few places on earth. The unique ecosystem of Upper Klamath Lake, Klamath Falls, Oregon is one of those unique places. The lake is rich in volcanic ash, minerals and pristine water.

SUPER BLUE GREEN ALGAE (SBGA)

Aphanizomenon Flos-Aquae is more commonly referred to as wild blue-green microalgae or AFA. This naturally abundant, premium wild-crafted organic microalgae contains a vast array of micronutrients such as the pigments chlorophyll, phycocyanin, beta-carotene, essential fatty acids, active enzymes, vitamins, all the essential amino acids, as well as minerals, trace minerals, proteins, complex sugars and other phytonutrients.

BLUE-GREEN MICROALGAE NUTRITIONAL CHART

Vitamins		Minerals & Trace Elements	
Vitamin E	Thiamin B1	Calcium	Molybdenum
Folic Acid	Riboflavin B2	Chloride	Phosphorus
Vitamin K	Pyridoxine B6	Chromium	Potassium
Biotin	Cobalamin B12	Copper	Selenium
Niacin	Pantothenic Acid	Iron	Sodium
Choline	Provitamin A	Magnesium	Zinc
Vitamin C	(beta-carotene)	Manganese	

Pigments & Other Nutrients		Essential Fatty Acids	
Chlorophyll	Beta-Carotene	Alpha-Linolenic Acid (Omega-3)	
Phenylethylamine	Canthaxanthin	Linoleic Acid (Omega-6)	
Phycocyanin	Glutathione		

Gram for gram this unique organic blue-green microalgae offers a greater variety of naturally health promoting micronutrients than any other food on earth.

This superfood helps me to increase:
- Energy, vitality, endurance
- Strengthens my immune system which fights disease
- Increase my mental performance, improves alertness and attention

- Supports brain function and the ability to manage my stress
- Supplies essential fatty acids, proteins, complex sugars, vitamins, minerals and amino acids
- High concentration of chlorophyll stimulates liver function and the excretion of bile, detoxifies chemical pollutants out of the body

I just love how great it makes me feel. I just mix a little powder in some water and take it to the gym at workout time.

STEMPLEX

Stemplex is a unique combination of natural ingredients that have been found to work synergistically to support the growth of adult stem cells.
- Increases the growth of adult stem cells as shown in vitro laboratory studies.
- Supports the body's natural renewal system through a unique combination of ingredients:
    - Green Tea helps support normal cholesterol levels, the digestive and respiratory systems, and healthy skin tissue.
    - Wild Blueberry supports the health of brain, heart, urinary tracts, eyes and normal glucose levels.
    - Carnosine is an antioxidant amino acid naturally present in the human body helps delay the natural aging of cells and extends the lifespan of adult stem cells.
    - Vitamin D supports adult stem cell renewal and helps these cells become immune cells for naturally fighting infections.

- o <u>Omega Sun</u> with patented wild AFA (SBGA), which increases the efficiency of the Stemplex formula.
- Provides nutrition that enables stem cells to flourish.
- Protects existing stem cells from the harmful effects of free radicals.

ESSENTIALS

The essentials pack makes using the organic super foods from Simplexity very easy and provides supplemental digestive enzymes and friendly flora. It contains 6 veggie caps: 2 super blue green algae, 2 enzymes and 2 probiotics. It's great to just throw in my purse or overnight bag for super food on the road.

LIFEGIVE SUPPLEMENTS FROM HHI

LifeGive supplements are formulated by and made exclusively for the world by renowned Hippocrates Health Institute. With their mission statement "Help People Help Themselves," Drs. Brian and Anna Marie Clement have created cutting edge whole food supplements. These supplements are made from plants and whole foods processed at low temperatures to preserve their heat sensitive enzymes and nutrients. These supplements are easily absorbed and assimilated by the body, and packaged carefully to ensure the life and bioavailability remains intact.

LifeGive supplements contain no: chemicals, preservatives, pesticides, herbicides, or fungicides, fillers, allergens, soy, dairy, corn, gluten, starch, no animal products. 100% Vegan Vegetarian.

My favorite daily supplements are:

1. HHI – Zymes - Contain all the digestive enzymes, essential nutrients, vitamins and minerals to enhance digestion of your meals. Taken 30 minutes before meals, especially important to be taken before cooked foods whose own enzymes have been destroyed by the heating above 118°F.
2. Phyto – Tumeric - powerful anti-cancer whole food supplement with active "curcuminoids", also increase brain function and contains anti-inflammatory properties.
3. Pinnacle - comprehensive thyroid complex promotes healthy thyroid function, detoxification of heavy metals, chemical toxins, helps reduce toxic effects of radiation treatments and chronic stress. Supports healthy metabolic rate.
4. Systemic Enzymes – supports healthy circulation, relieves oxidative stress, and facilitates quick recovery after exercise. Contains proprietary enzyme blend plus Vitamin C, calcium, ginger, rutin, and grape seed extract. To be taken between meals.

CHIA SEEDS

Chia seeds should be raw and ground, 100% organic. Virtually lost for 500 years, this ancient Aztec seed was once a dietary mainstay. Chia's resurgence into the 21st century marketplace could potentially alleviate the nutritional health concerns of millions. Chia seeds may contain the highest amount of omega 3's in the plant world.

Today we know (or we should know) the importance of "good" fat in our diets. The alpha linolenic fatty acid (ALA) found in Chia seeds are known as the only essential omega-3 fatty acid which must be consumed as the human body cannot make it. Omega-3 is also found in olive oil, flax seed, flax oil and a few others, but can go rancid very quickly if not consumed shortly after pressing or grinding. It should be kept refrigerated or frozen. Chia seeds do not go rancid so you can always be sure that you are consuming a good fungus-free source of omega-3. Chia seeds are a great source of protein (the building blocks of your body, hair, skin, nails, muscles, red blood cells, etc.), both essential and non-essential amino acids and fiber which is necessary for a healthy heart and good circulation. It also modulates blood sugar and helps fill you up (so can eat less empty unhealthy calories) while providing antioxidants and phytonutrients, these two essential components to human health. Interestingly they are not absolutely necessary for life. We can drag along without them for years, never feeling really good but just surviving until some disease overtakes us.

Gram for gram Chia seeds contain:
8x more Omega 3 than salmon
6x more calcium than milk
3x more iron than spinach
15x more magnesium than broccoli
2x more fiber than bran flakes
6x more protein than kidney beans
4x more phosphorus than whole milk
More antioxidants than blueberries

Chia seeds are so packed with nutritional benefits that it is being touted as the "world's healthiest whole food". I consume 1-2 Tbs every day just to cover all my nutritional bases.

CHAPTER 27

⌘

WEIMAR-NEW START PROGRAM

I decided to go to Weimar Institute after attending a 3 week juicing program in Washington State run by Seventh Day Adventists. It was here that I first heard about Weimar's nutritional program.

Studies conducted at Loma Linda University, John Hopkins, Harvard just to name a few wanted to learn why the vegan-vegetarian lifestyle of the Seventh Day Adventist Church members had reduced their risk of Type II Diabetes, strokes, heart attacks, fibromyalgia, cancer, osteoporosis, arthritis, most diseases associated with high blood pressure, high cholesterol, blood sugar imbalances, hormone imbalances, and many other chronic diseases. Pretty amazing. Not only did they live an average of 10 years longer, but the quality of their health was so much better.

After finishing my Hippocrates Health Educator Program I realized one thing. Many guests that I met at Hippocrates seemed unable, unwilling or both to stick to a completely living, raw food diet.

An Alumni session of the usual 3 week New Start Program was coming up so I asked one of the doctors at Weimar if I could attend. I was there for five days. I figured nothing I ate in five days could be that harmful to my body. So I temporarily abandoned my wheatgrass, juicing and raw "living" food protocols.

I was amazed at what I saw in the 5 day session. The Alumni were vibrant and full of success stories. It was so much fun. Everything and everyone seemed so relaxed and easy.

N	Nutrition
E	Exercise
W	Water
S	Sunshine
T	Temperance
A	Air
R	Rest
T	Trust

Nutrition

Bible based nutrition, more details can be found in Ellen G. White's book <u>Counsel on Diet and Foods</u>: whole grains, fruits, nuts, seeds, and vegetables prepared in as simple and natural a manner as possible. Eat organically or locally grown foods (more nutrition), avoid all processed, refined foods, choose foods whose types of nutrients will improve circulation, strengthen immune system and reduce cholesterol in the body.

Allowed foods include:
- All fruit, preferably fresh, but also frozen (unsweetened), or canned in fruit juice or water packed
- All greens, especially turnip greens, mustard greens, radish greens, collards, kale, broccoli, or cabbage. Use sparingly high oxalate foods such as spinach, chard, or beet greens, peanuts, or rhubarb
- All herbs that are mild
- All legumes (beans, peas, lentils, and garbanzos) etc.
- All whole grains. You need two kinds daily plus a legume or greens to get optimal balance of amino acids
- Nuts in moderation. The better ones are the non-

tropical nuts such as almonds, filberts, pecans, and walnuts. Use no peanut butter or peanuts

No animal products:
- No flesh foods--meat, fish, or fowl
- No egg yolks
- No milk products--milk, cheese, or butter

Eat no refined foods:
- No oil, margarine, shortening
- No sugar, syrup, or free starch
- No white bread, white rice
- No degerminated corn meal
- No gluten or soy
- No meat substitutes or powdered soy milk

All nutritional needs, daily serving, should include:
- 2 fruits
- 2 cups yellow and green vegetables
- A steamed legume such as beans, peas, lentils
- 2-3 types whole grains
- B12 vitamin chewed with food weekly
- Kelp tablet daily (for iodine) if salt restricted

Guests on restricted diets for heart disease, arthritis, or diabetes should reduce intake of nuts, seeds, olives, avocado, soy beans and tofu.

Rules for good digestion: eat slowly, chew your food 30-40 times per mouthful to mix with your saliva. Don't drink with meals it dilutes process of proper digestion. Eat two meals per day. Evening meal can be skipped or light soup, fruit and bread. Eat a variety of vegetables, whole grains, potatoes and fruit, but limit to 4-5 types of any one during a meal. Limit salt intake. Flavor foods with lemon, onion, mild spices, and herbs. Do not overcook, over clean, peel too much to retain essential vitamins, minerals, and trace elements.

Breakfast at Weimar consisted of generous amounts of whole grain cereals (oatmeal, millet, cornmeal mush, granola in many delicious flavors) served with fresh almond milk or soy milk. Delicious fruits (bananas, cherries, blueberries, strawberries, melons), soy (tofu) based gravy over homemade biscuits, lots of homemade breads and almond butter.

Lunch was the main meal of the day. Lots of raw fresh salad with two types of dressings. The house dressing was my favorite almost like a creamy ranch dressing made of raw cashews and tofu. There was always a cooked entree of beans, brown rice, yams, steamed vegetables like bell peppers, onions, garlic, squash, kale, chard, collard greens, veggie burgers, tofu based stews, and again fresh baked breads, crackers with hummus, and a few types of fruit.

Dinner (supper) was a light soup, some salad greens, fresh bread, and a little fruit.

Exercise

Exercise a minimum of 20-30 minutes at your best level of endurance at least five days a week. Walking is good exercise. The New Start Program mantra is "walk, walk, walk." Get plenty of outdoor walking on the 15 plus miles of outdoor trails in the foothills of the Sierra Nevada Mountains above Auburn, California.

Some interesting facts:
- "50% of heart disease, stroke, yes even cancer would be reduced with regular exercise," Dr. Kenneth Cooper of the Aerobics Center Texas
- Exercise is the only permanent weight loss solution.
- 60% of Americans are considered sedentary, 55% are overweight.

- Eating free (refined) fats turns on the cholesterol mechanism in the liver. Free fats are absorbed high in the gut and are dumped into the heart. Oil in plant fiber is absorbed lower and the liver processes it before it circulates through to the heart.

Water

The body needs water for internal and external cleansing. Drink six to eight glasses of water daily, more if you sweat a lot. Drink water on rising, between meals, but early enough before bedtime to avoid interrupting sleep to urinate. Drinking water during exercise increases endurance.

Sunshine

You need at least 10 minutes of sunshine every day. Vitamin D can be stored in your body for weeks. Avoid burning.

Temperance

Eliminate all tea, coffee, soft-drinks, and alcoholic beverages from your diet. Drink filtered or distilled water. Use moderation in all things. Particularly do not overeat.

Air

Get fresh air with negatively ionized particles from forests, lakes, and oceans when possible. Breathe deeply as part of your walking program when possible.

Rest

Get plenty of sleep. Don't eat too much for supper. Overeating causes your body to slow digestion when sleeping. It can also keep you awake. Avoid stressful situations, relax in a warm tub.

Trust in God

Faith in a loving Master will help you rest physically and mentally.

Included at Weimar are wonderful varieties of massage and hydrotherapies, hyperthermia treatment and hot and cold foot and tub therapies. I felt so good after my treatments and massages. So relaxed.

Every meal the doctors were available to discuss your problems or just chat. They also joined the patients on hikes and were very available at their clinic all week. I was impressed with their depth of knowledge and everything they discussed was backed with extensive research material. Every day lectures were given on different health topics. There were always heated discussions about milk, beef, chicken... they pulled out there research materials and stuck to the facts.

I highly recommend Weimar's New Start Program. The vigorous hiking in lush mountains was great for me. The fresh air was so invigorating. The prayer and meditation kept me centered and balanced. The food was delicious, I forgot about proper food combining about the third day. All that good exercise seemed to keep things digesting just fine.

I again feel so blessed to have had the opportunity to go to this very special place. I feel now that I have some healthy alternative cooked foods that I can offer as suggestions to clients and friends who find the totally raw food diet to be too restrictive and difficult for them to maintain. The nutritious Weimar recipes can, I believe, help people "bridge the gap" between the two different nutritional philosophies.

For cancer patients I think at least 80% raw, organic, sprouted, living foods is imperative. Fruits and fats feed hungry cancer cells. Precious vitamin C is lost in cooking. Just doing your research is an essential part of nutrition. The road to recovery and full remission from cancer requires incredible focus and discipline, particularly in the beginning as you are probably coming from the Standard American Diet (SAD).

Contact information New Start Lifestyle Program call 800-525-9192 or www.NewStart.com

CHAPTER 28
⌘
HIPPOCRATES HEALTH INSTITUTE NOURISHMENT FOR THE MIND-BODY-SPIRIT

I traveled to Hippocrates Health Institute in West Palm Beach, Florida to try to answer the question "I'm a vegan now so what should I eat?" I never dreamed how much it would change my life.

The first contact I had with raw food vegans (vegans eat no animals or products from animals, no fish) was at a conference in Florida put together by a wonderful man named John Eagle Freedom. I heard informative lectures by T. Collin Campbell (<u>The China Study</u>), Victorus Kulvinskus (<u>Survival in the 21st Century</u>), Drs. Brian and Anna Marie Clement (<u>Longevity</u>, <u>Supplements Exposed</u>, <u>Toxic Clothing</u>). During the conference raw food chefs Jackie and Gideon Graff prepared the most delicious raw food lunch and dinner dishes I had ever eaten. After my four days of eating raw foods twice a day I knew that something wonderful was happening in my body. I began to feel a little extra "pep" in my step. I could think more clearly.

Dr. Lubecki was also one of the keynote speakers. He met with Drs. Brian and Anna Maria Clement after his presentation and they decided to fly to California to get more information on Dr. Lubecki's amazing treatment protocols.

After spending three days in California with Dr. Lubecki, they decided to bring his entire protocol to their world renowned Hippocrates Health Institute back in West Palm Beach, Florida. We flew to their facility a few weeks later. It was definitely the most luxurious "swimming pools and movie stars…"and comprehensive health facility that I had ever been to in all my travels.

Dr. Lubecki treated at least sixty guests and close to all of the staff. During his presentation he shocked everyone when he interrupted the French interpreter and spoke to that group and several others in their native languages. I believe Dr. Lubecki, a very humble man, speaks about seven languages. Dr. Lubecki tirelessly saw guests and staff from 9:00am to 9:00pm every day. He then rejuvenated under the big laser and was ready to begin again. We swam one night at 11:00pm and then fell to sleep in our luxurious townhouse on the property. At 80 years young he never ceases to amaze me. His kindness, humility and breadth of knowledge is overwhelming. His devotion to his patients is only surpassed by his devotion to God. He believes that God is the source of all his inspiration and guidance in helping people heal themselves.

It was then and there that I decided that I needed to go through the Hippocrates Health Educator program and bring the Hippocrates raw "living" foods protocols back to Dr. Lubecki's patients. Proper lifestyle and nutrition are important keys to prevention and treatment of cancer and other diseases.

I spent the next nine weeks usually 10-12 hours per day learning exactly what it means to be a Hippocrates Health Educator. It would take me sixteen volumes to explain it all to you. The best source of information would be to go through the program yourself; otherwise, I suggest going to the three week Lifestyle Program.

3 WEEK LIFESTYLE PROGRAM
(Excerpts from Lifestyle Program DVD)

Hippocrates has about 60 new guests each week. The

grounds are filled with exotic plants, and so many little hidden spots for guests to meditate or talk privately. It is truly a spiritual sanctuary. The staff teach and live the Living Foods Lifestyle which focuses on a diet of organic living, raw foods: such as sprouts, green juices, vegetables, sea vegetables, soaked and sprouted grains, nuts and seeds. Staff and guests drink wheatgrass juice, a powerful cleansing and healing agent that enhances the healing process.

Hippocrates is not just a health center, but also a health school showing how live foods and increased oxygen improve the state of your health. Tests have proven that enzymes and oxygen nourishment from raw living foods help the body to correct any imbalances or weaknesses that cause illness. You will literally rebuild your health.

The institute was started in 1955 by Ann Wigmore who healed herself of cancer. She wanted to share her knowledge with people who wanted to heal themselves naturally.

In addition to the living foods diet, Hippocrates designs a personalized program for each guest, including analysis of their blood – with regular blood tests as well as darkfield microscopy. Proper food supplements are recommended and different protocols are suggested. Free analysis of guests' blood test results are given for two years after the 3 week program ends.

They teach you the importance of exercise and rest, and also help you heal emotional wounds. Thousands of people have healed themselves by giving their bodies the proper nutrition needed by every cell and by eliminating the toxins that create disease. We know that our immune systems have been designed impeccably just that no one gave us an owner's manual for the proper care and feeding of your body.

Hippocrates goes to work to educate their guests to help create that "owners manual". Guests are given daily lectures by Drs. Brian and Anna Marie Clement, as well as staff and outside lecturers with impressive credentials. Subjects are thoroughly covered on: basic health principles and the benefits of the raw, living foods lifestyle; detoxification and elimination; proper food combining; the importance of fasting on green juices one day per week; whole food supplementation, fresh water algae's, AFA (blue green) and chlorella (green); ancient remedies – wheatgrass poultices, garlic oil treatments, cayenne pepper for blood loss; herbs as medicine; homeopathy; sprouting; soaking and sprouting nuts and seeds; dehydration and food prep classes; skin care and cosmetics that are healthy; far infrared sauna benefits; hand held and large lasers health benefits; importance of dry skin brushing before showering; lymphatic massage; proper spinal alignment; exercise including Yoga, Tai Chi, swimming, weight lifting, rebounding are thoroughly explained and available daily for the guests; meditation, psychotherapy, hypnotherapy, art therapy, compassionate communication methods and the importance of the mind-body-spirit connection; growing your own wheatgrass and other sprouts classes are available at their own greenhouse; journaling; importance of rest... the list is endless.

Each guest receives a 2' binder outlining classes and subject materials and extra paper for taking notes. Guests are encouraged to attend the lectures, but no one is ever forced to do anything.

When guests are not in classes or doing therapies they can enjoy mineral pools, ozonated pools and spas, cold pool (very cold for dipping 7 times to increase circulation), steam saunas, Far infrared saunas, sit by running streams or numerous fountains, or just talk and enjoy other guest's companionship and success stories. Music fills the air on dance nights, Dr. Brian Clement is the drummer in the "Wheatgrass Band" (which is very good). When he is not on a speaking tour he will entertain the guests with music from the 60's, 70's, 80's eras. Guests look forward to this night almost as much as frozen banana or nut ice cream night once a week.

In addition to all the numerous free treatments, Hippocrates also offers individualized counseling sessions with licensed psychologists and hypnotherapist, hyperbaric oxygen therapies, aqua chi footbath with a metatronic electrical stimulator detox therapy, hydrocolon therapy, several types of massages, biofeedback, Hwave pain therapy, various oxygen therapies, it is quite extensive and impressive.

I will give you some of the bare bone basics now. The raw food vegan lifestyle restores balance within the body. Fresh, raw "living" foods nourish, alkalize, and cleanse the body. As Thomas Edison said, "The doctor of the future will give no medicine but will interest his patients in the care of the human frame in diet and in the cause and prevention of disease."

1. WATER
Drink one half of your body weight in ounces of fresh, clean water every day. Many people suffer from dehydration at the cellular level. By the time you are thirsty you are already very dehydrated. Coffee, soda, and sweet fruit juices do not count toward your necessary water intake. In fact caffeine in coffee and soda actually dehydrates the body more.

2. WHEATGRASS JUICE
Wheatgrass juice, drink two to four ounces of freshly squeezed per day. One ounce of wheatgrass juice contains 103 vitamins, minerals and amino acids. It represents as much nutritional value as 2 ½ pounds of fresh green vegetables. Wheatgrass is high in chlorophyll. It is a natural source of B-17 laetrile (known cancer fighter), A, B

complex, C, E, and K. Wheatgrass contains beta-carotene (also found in red, green, yellow pigmented fruits and vegetables). It cleanses, purifies and nourishes the body by activating white blood cells which boosts the immune system thereby destroying free radicals in the body from ingested toxins, air pollution, cigarette smoke… the list of damaging free radicals is endless. As a natural blood cleanser it increases enzyme levels, builds red blood cells, aids digestion, and regenerates the liver. It's also great for weight loss and pets.

Wheatgrass should be consumed on an empty stomach for maximum benefit.

Wheatgrass is easiest in the morning, wait 15-30 minutes before eating for proper absorption. Start slowly, build up to 2 ounces in the morning and 2 ounces in the evening 1 ½-3 hours after eating. Digestion begins in your mouth with salivary glands so try to swish it around in your mouth before swallowing. Wheatgrass can be purchased at many stores. Wheatgrass shots are offered at juice bars. Fresh cut wheatgrass can be stored in plastic containers for up to seven days. Store it dry.

Debbie's green bags (now in many brands) store all vegetables longer and keep it fresher than just leaving it in the tray crisper or plastic bags.

Chlorophyll contains so many elements that it is called nature's greatest healer. It is made from sunlight because it is the "blood" of plants. Its molecular structure is almost identical to the hemoglobin molecule of human blood. Wheatgrass is a superior form of chlorophyll. Wheatgrass when grown in organic soil absorbs over 100 elements needed by our bodies.

3. DETOXIFICATION

Detoxification of the body can be greatly enhanced by

incorporating 1-2 ounces of wheatgrass juice in your enema bag or 4 ounces in a rectal implant after a fresh water enema. It cleanses the colon and stimulates internal organs. It is great for constipation. Enemas and wheatgrass implants are an integral part of the program, done twice per day.

4. GREEN DRINKS

Green drinks are mixtures of freshly squeezed juices. 50% sprouts and 50% vegetables is the ideal combination. Ideally you should drink at least two glasses per day. I use a Green Star twin auger juicer. First I juice my wheatgrass 2 ounces (more if I'm doing an enema or implant) then I wait 30 minutes and make my morning green drink. My recipe consists of one handful of pea shoots, one handful of sunflower sprouts, one cucumber, 3-4 stalks of celery (this is Hippocrates Green Drink), then I throw in whatever I have, kale, parsley, arugula, romaine lettuce, red bell pepper, dandelion greens, 2 cloves of garlic, a small piece of ginger, and turmeric, mung bean sprouts, parsley, asparagus, daikon root, or cabbage. Find out what works for you but try to drink this at a bare minimum of once daily within 15 minutes of juicing it to maximum enzymes and nutrients.

To simplify the process I usually juice shop one day per week. I use the green bags and put all the ingredients for a juice in the same bag. Example-3 stalks celery, 2 kale leaves, ½ cucumber, ½ red bell pepper, 4" chunk daikon root, 8 dandelion leaves, handful of arugula, spinach, pea shoots, sunflower sprouts, mung bean shoots, use chard or collard green leaf if no kale is available. I wash it on the day that I use it. It stores much better if it's dry. Always put a non-chlorinated paper towel in the bag to soak up extra moisture; I keep the mung beans separate as too much moisture gets in the bag. **Side note: kale and arugula are very high in nutrients. Try to juice them every day if possible or eat them in your salads.**

5. PROPER FOOD COMBINING

Food combining is difficult to do but really aids in proper digestion. The following charts help explain. Don't drink 30 minutes before meals or 2-3 hours afterwards this keeps your digestive juices from becoming diluted.

GOOD COMBINATIONS	POOR COMBINATIONS
Avocado & Greens	Fruit & Starch
Avocado & Sub-acid fruit	Fruit & Vegetable
Protein & Sprouts and Leafy Greens	Fruit & Protein
Starch & Sprouts & Vegetables	Starch & Protein
	Starch & Avocado

PROTEINS 4HRS	CARBO/STARCHES 2-3HRS
Nuts, (almonds, pecans, walnuts, etc.)	Sprouted Grains (wheat, rye, etc.)
Seeds (pumpkin, sesame, sunflower, etc.)	Sprouted Beans (chickpeas, etc.)
	Sprouted Peas, Winter squash
	Potato (juice)

Protein and Starchy Carbohydrates - When taken together create over 120 chemicals in the body, most notably sulfur, stops digestion and pollutes the blood. About 50% of health problems can be linked to poor combinations. Protein (4hrs to digest) is best eaten in the afternoon when you have the most hydrochloric acid in your digestive tract. Starchy Carbohydrates (2 1/2 hrs to digest) are the best eaten in evening.

Fruit – Organic and ripe. Insecticide sprayed 15x more often on fruit. At best healthy people/children should have no more than 15% of diet fruit due to its high fructose from hybridization.

> **ACID FRUIT**
> **1 TO 1 1/2HRS**
> Lemons
> Oranges
> Grapefruit
> Pineapple
> Strawberries

Acid – Citrus, pineapple, strawberries

> **SUB-ACID FRUIT**
> **1 ½ TO 2HRS**
> Apples, Pears
> Grapes, Peaches
> Sweet Cherries
> Apricots
> Berries (most)

> **SWEET FRUIT**
> **3 TO 4HRS(IF RIPE)**
> Bananas
> Dried Fruit (Figs, dates, raisins, etc.)
> Persimmons

SubAcid – Cherries, mangoes, apples, peaches, pears, and tomatoes.

<u>Sweet</u> – Dried fruit. **Unripened fruit robs the body of minerals.** It's best to eat one fruit at a time.

```
┌─────────────────────────────┐
│         AVOCADO             │
│        45 MIN-2HRS          │
│   ───────────────────       │
│      Combines well with:    │
│          Acid Fruit         │
│        Sub-acid Fruit       │
│        Leafy Greens         │
└─────────────────────────────┘
```

```
┌──────────────────────────────────────────────┐
│                 VEGETABLES                     │
│                   2-3HRS                        │
│   ──────────────────────────────────────       │
│  Sprouted Greens (alfalfa, sunflower, buckwheat,│
│            lentils, mung, etc.)                 │
│  Leafy Greens, Celery, Cucumber, Beets, Carrots │
│              (mildly starchy)                    │
│  Summer Squash, Sweet Pepper, Asparagus,        │
│          Fresh Corn, Fresh Peas                 │
└──────────────────────────────────────────────┘
```

Fruit and vegetables should never be consumed together. They have different enzymes which are incompatible in the body. They go through the digestive tract at different times. Avocado, garlic, onions, and edible flowers can be eaten with fruit or vegetables.

```
┌─────────────────────────────────┐
│           MELONS                │
│          15-30MIN               │
│  ─────────────────────────────  │
│  (Melons are always eaten alone) │
│  Cantaloupes, Crenshaw, Honeydew,│
│           Watermelon            │
│  (When juicing use entire fruit │
│         including rind)         │
└─────────────────────────────────┘
```

Melons – Eaten alone or left alone can be mixed with each other only. They are about 85% water and very high in sugar.

Your stomach is a holding tank first in first out, in our digestive track. You eat protein (4 hours to digest) with carbohydrates (2-3 hours) and top it off with a great piece of melon (15-30 minutes) you will start a nasty fermentation process. Digestion will stop, the decomposing foods just sit fermenting in the digestive system. Cancer loves this composting environment. It has a feeding frenzy.

6. DIET ESSENTIALS

Sprouts - 10x to 30x more nutritious than mature vegetables. Edible and nutritious land based food all create alkalinity. 1lb of seed becomes 10lbs of nutritious food – could wipe out world hunger. 5000 types of edible seeds could become edible sprouts. Wheatgrass and sunflower sprouts highest chlorophyll and give you tons of energy. Wheatgrass juice is used for wound healing.

```
╭─────────────────────────────╮
│      WHEATGRASS              │
│      15-30 MIN              │
│  ─────────────────────────  │
│  Use only on empty stomach or│
│  before meals. Extract juice by│
│     chewing or juicing.     │
│  Use alone or with other green│
│      vegetable juices.      │
╰─────────────────────────────╯
```

Clover, radish, broccoli, chia, onion sprouts contain ½ chlorophyll of wheatgrass. 2 green drinks per day. Onion and garlic sprouts are good purifiers. Fenugreek is a healing sprout. Its gel is very good for diabetic wounds. If gets rid of bacteria. It also eliminates body odor.

Sea Vegetables - Raw form – most nutrition from ocean, richest mineral source (wakami, dulse, and nori are very good).

Fresh Water Algaes - Most nutritious food from fresh water. Positively changes DNA and helps the body build new stem cells. Should be taken as a supplement forever. First life form on earth.

Blue Green (AFA) – Klamath Lake has high mineral vortex water and has no hard shell around algae. Very easy to digest.

Green – Chlorella – Japanese have cracked open the hard shell for easier digestion.

Most people are sick and unhealthy because people are eating too much dead (cooked) foods and processed foods loaded with chemicals and preservatives. These people have never even heard of fresh water algaes and their amazing healing properties.

Grains – Millet, buckwheat, amaranth, quinoa, teff (soak for 6 hours – drain and rinse 2x per day, sprouts in 2 days) very alkalizing grains for building body and energy producers.

Beans – Lots of roughage. Helps relieve atrophy in digestive tract which causes gas. 17x-57x more digestible if soaked and sprouted first. Pinto 27x more digestible, kidney 57x more digestible. High quality proteins for energy. **Soybeans and black beans don't eat due to hybridization, changes molecule structure hard to digest.** Mung and adzuki beans should be grown in total darkness. Mung beans need to be sprouted under pressure. A plate on top of strainer will do. They are high in minerals; also help fight prostate and breast cancer.

Herbs – 80% of the world uses herbs. They are medicine and should not be taken long term. Asian herbs are the most documented.

7. THERE ARE FOUR FACTS ABOUT CANCER

- Cancer cannot live in an alkaline environment. The body has to neutralize your pH to restore your body's perfect balance. You cannot live if your body becomes too acidic. Changing your diet is the number one key to proper alkalinity. Drugs, processed foods, most sugars, and white rice are very acidic.

- Cancer cannot live in an oxygenated environment. Raw "living" foods - sunflower, sprouts, and wheatgrass are loaded with chlorophyll which is extremely oxygenating. Hyperbaric chambers and ozone therapies are also great. Exercise with oxygen is also used in many health facilities.

- Cancer cannot survive in high levels of enzymes. Certain digestive enzymes eat the cancer cell's protective coating. A raw "living" food plant based diet is the highest source of enzymes from foods. Also, whole food enzyme supplementation should be considered. Both digestive and systemic enzymes are

the "workforce" of the body.   Nothing gets done
without them.
- Cancer cannot live if heated above 104-105°.   Several
  treatments are available that heat the body.   Far
  infrared sauna is used extensively for this treatment.
  Hyperthermia is another common treatment to raise
  the body's temperature.

8. WHOLE FOOD VITAMIN SUPPLEMENTATION

New ERA of HOPE came in with Dr. Lee's work with
whole food supplementation.   People were becoming
malnourished as the industrial age started depleting the
soil of necessary minerals, fast food, canned food, and
packaged foods killed important nutrients and enzymes.
Dr. Lee was able to maintain the vitamins, herbs, proteins,
minerals and enzymes of whole foods while drying and
compressing them into capsule form.   These whole food
supplements are Bio Active (live) and easily absorbable by
the body.   Best of all recognized by the body as food not
synthetic, made in laboratories isolated vitamins and
minerals that your immune system starts to attack because
it sees it as a foreign substance not good for the body.

Below are some of the components in organic, raw, whole
food supplementation.
H Hormones
O Oxygen
P Phytochemicals
E Enzymes

The Hippocrates whole food supplements are particularly
important for people with compromised immune systems.
In a two year study of Ill and Well patients, the Ill group
had better immune recovery 26% more from whole food

supplementation, the already <u>Well</u> group has 7% increased immune system recovery. Fabulous numbers. Healing takes time. For an <u>Ill</u> person to get to the same immune system level as the <u>Well</u> person took about two years on various necessary supplementation. Four other things were also necessary to regain fully functioning immune systems:

100% organic raw living foods diet
Exercise
Positive Attitude
Spiritual Connection

9. <u>FASTING</u>

Juice fasting should be done 1 day per week. 1 day/week = 52 days/year (no water fasting - unnecessarily hard on body). Juice should be 50% sprouts and 50% organic vegetables. Hippocrates uses their organic green drink - sprouts, 1/2 sunflower sprouts or 1/2 pea shoots (about 4 cups), 3-4 stalks of celery, 1/2 cucumber, spinach, parsley, kale. Drink fresh wheatgrass juice - 2oz morning/evening. Drink fresh cucumber juice 9:00am. Drink green drink 11:00/12:30 (lunch) and 4:00pm. Green drink soup - made with green drink and avocado mixture - very satisfying.
Fasting helps put the human experience more in balance. The body has three centers:
Head - Mental, spiritual: Understanding of your part in the universe.
Heart - Emotional: Understanding of self. All there is in life is change - learn to be lover of change. Need clearer vision of self - fasting helps bring this about.
Physical - Sexual (male/female); Food - oxygen, water, nourishment; Exercise (getting heart rate going 30 minutes/5 days/week) - Aerobics, weight lifting 3/week

for 1 hour, yoga; Rest - At 50 years old you need 8-8 1/2 hours per night, at 80 years old you need 6 1/2 hours per night, not enough sleep you can actually lose hours off your lifespan, sleep deprivation causes loss of mental acuity; Sunshine - Before 9:00am after 4:00pm best to avoid wrinkles and skin damage; Physical brain - Neurologically ready to be hit by the next shockwave of fear, anger, or hostility.

We should use these three centers equally: 1/3, 1/3, 1/3 instead our energy gets anchored to the bottom. Digesting food, fasting helps crack the eggshell of physical, so to speak, to allow the energy to flow upward to other centers of the body. Right now only imbalance in centers 91% of all human energy stuck in bottom center: physical: sex, food, hate, fear, anxiety. 8% in middle center: emotional - How can I become happy, joyful - <1% top center: mental/spiritual - Renaissance in spirituality will come only with balance.

Fasting after 2/3 months will begin process of cleansing, restoring health, improving/faster thought patterns, improving brain overall functioning, getting clearer vision of self, better self-esteem.

SUMMARY

We are all striving for love and happiness. Putting our life in its proper perspective in the universe will bring us all closer to the "Greater Good Community of Mankind" that I can see off in the distance.

I saved Hippocrates Health Institute for the end of my book because I thought it was important to end with the lifestyle I choose to embrace. I am not there yet. I still have trouble giving up some favorite cooked foods. As I learn more dehydrated foods I'm sure I can soon reach my goal. I never chastise myself, I just figure I'll do more raw foods tomorrow.

Hippocrates Health Institute is now my favorite vacation destination. I loved the staff, the friends I call my Class of 2011 Hippocrates Health Educators (three of whom I now call best friends), the food was delicious, the classes were life changing. Thank you to Drs. Brian and Anna Marie Clement for your depth of knowledge, grace, and love for what you choose to do with your lives. It shines through as you greet every guest like a best friend.

For more information contact:
Susan Gorkosky
Hippocrates Health Educator
info@juicingforcancer.com

RECOMMENDED READING

During the past three years I have done some extensive reading in my continuing search for vibrant health. Below is a short list of books that I consider particularly helpful. They are on different aspects of health and equally important.

Because People Are Dying, The Story of a Rock, An Apple and Cancer, by Jane G. Goldberg, PHD., Sea Raven Press, 2009
This book discusses Radiation Hormesis, the studies, science and research behind the healing powers of the radioactive stones used by Jay Gutierrez. Low dose radiation stones and mud packs should be in your arsenal of tools for incredible pain relief and healing. I cannot imagine a night of deep, restful sleep without my mud packs. There is an incredible amount of research behind the powerful pain relief I get from these stones. Jay can be reached at www.nighthawkminerals.com.

The China Study, by T. Colin Campbell, PhD., Ben Bella Books, Inc., 2006
This is the most comprehensive study ever done on the negative effects of animal protein on the human body. This study is one of the most convincing arguments for a plant-based diet. The study strongly supports the fact that a vegetarian diet helps prevent a broad range of diseases: heart disease, obesity, type 2 diabetes, breast cancer, colon cancer, prostate cancer, MS and other autoimmune diseases, just to name a few.
This book has been on the New York Times bestseller list since its publication in 2006. Get it - Read it.
One very interesting study involving rats is especially shocking. A group of several hundred rats were given aflatoxin (a cancer causing fungus found on peanuts and

corn). It is highly carcinogenic and used on lab rats to induce cancerous tumors). Rats generally live two years. This was a one hundred week study. All the rats that were given the aflatoxin and fed 20% casein (animal protein consisting of 7% cow's milk) were dead from liver cancer at 100 weeks. The other rats given the aflatoxin and only 5% casein were alive, active, sleek hair coat and no sign of liver cancer - Score 100-0. Some of the rats that were fed the 20% casein were switched at forty or sixty weeks to 5% casein (animal protein) 35-40 % had reversed their cancer growth. Rats switched from 5% to 20% animal protein started growing full blown cancer tumors. Study findings indicated that cancer could be turned on and off through nutritional manipulation. The actual "China Study" involved 24 of the 27 provinces of China and 6,500 people, many variables and decades of research. Fascinating reading. Be prepared, you will never look at that glass of cow's milk or steak the same way after this.

The Daylight Diet, Divine Eating for Superior Health and Digestion, by Paul Nison, 343 Publishing Co., 2009
I heard Paul Nison speak at the Health and Wealth Summit Conference in West Palm Beach, Florida. He is funny. I mean really funny. I felt like I was in a New York comedy club. His book reflects that same humor without detracting from his very important message. It is not only important to eat organic, raw "living" foods, but WHEN you eat them is every bit as critical. The old adage "Early to Bed, Early to Rise Makes a Man Healthy, Wealthy and Wise" comes to mind. His message: "eat during the daylight hours, eat less, and don't eat when you are stressed", Great recipes, enjoyable reading.

Detoxify or Die, by Sherry A. Rogers, M.D., Sand Key Company, Inc., 2002

Dr. Rogers writes a no nonsense, no holds barred book on environmental pollutants attacking our immune system on a daily basis. It's almost too much to take at times. What I really like about the book is that she presents the toxic pollutants, the tests to find out what toxins are hiding in our bodies and the various solutions to the toxic overload. It is by far the most comprehensive book on this subject that I have ever read. I consider it a "must read" if you want to maintain a healthy body.

Cancer-Free, Your Guide to Gentle, Non-Toxic Healing, by Bill Henderson, 3rd Edition, Booklocker, Inc., 2008

I met Bill Henderson two years ago at the convention put on by the Cancer Control Society in Southern California. His background is investigative journalism. After his wife's death from cancer in 1994, his life's work has been spent seeking out alternative treatments for cancer. Not the traditional "cut-burn-poison" approach. He now advocates Dr. Garcia's and Dr Lubecki's treatments and his interviews have convinced many people from all over the world to seek natural cures for chronic conditions. His web talk show called "How to live cancer free" has a listener base of over 50,000 people. You will find it at www.webtalkradio.net. Bill's book is filled with painstaking research and information on many good alternative cancer protocols.

Healing Light, Energy Medicine of the Future, by Larry Lytle, DDS, PhD., Author House, 2004

I have had the opportunity to spend the day with Dr. Lytle when he came out to see Dr. Lubecki. He holds 9 patents on the Q1000 technology. He is taking soft (cold) laser therapy to new heights. He is pushing the Q1000 laser and enhancers: 660 and 808 through the rigors of FDA testing and eventual approval, which is no small task. It takes a lot of money, time and effort to get anything into clinical trials with the FDA. I admire his tenacity and intelligence. In his book, <u>Healing Light</u>, he explains topics like Quantum Physics in a fairly easy to understand format. He reviews the Autonomic Nervous System, Dental Distress Syndrome & the Sympathetic and Parasympathetic Nervous Systems and the important role that dentistry plays in our pursuit of wellness. He calls dentistry the "missing link" of wellness. His explanation of the laser is in depth, research based and extremely helpful. His goal is to have a Q1000 in every home in America, as a first line of defense medical device: replacing pharmaceuticals like aspirin. It really works. I use my laser for everything every day. I can't imagine my life without it.

<u>The Healing Nature of Jesus</u>, by John Eagle Freedom & Susan Smith Jones, Healing Nature Press, 2010
This book is a goldmine of information, each chapter is written by a different dynamic published author and expert in their many different fields. Each chapter is a synopsis of the authors various books and life's work boiled down to a few pages. Loaded with information on diet, water, exercise, enzymes, living stress free, air pollution, cell phones, the list goes on. Another must read. I couldn't stop reading it; that's a lot to say for a book on health.

<u>The Healing Power of Water</u>, Dr. Masaru Emoto, Hay House Inc., 2007
Dr. Emoto was made famous by his studies and fabulous photography of water crystals in his book, <u>The Message From Water</u>. In the <u>Healing Power of Water</u>, he discusses how we can actually put a healing process into motion by thinking and feeling "love and gratitude". Since reading this book I write sayings and messages of love, gratitude, health, abundance and joy on all my bottles of water. I bless my water and thank

it and God for water's healing properties. The photography is so beautiful and his message is life changing.

Hippocrates, Life Force, Superior Health and Longevity, by Brian R. Clement, PhD, NMD, LNC, Healthy Living Publications, BPC, 2007

As the director of the world renowned Hippocrates Health Institute for over 30 years, Dr. Brian Clement has been a part of probably the largest on-going, real-life human research project exposing the rising benefits of the raw "living food" diet. His book goes into the nuts and bolts of the raw "living food" diet. The Hippocrates Health Institute has helped thousands of people with every imaginable disease. Raw "living foods", clean water, exercise, plenty of sunshine, proper supplementation, sleep, quiet time to pray & reflect and volunteer work to help others are all part of their formula for success. A great look at the different successes people have had as they change from the Standard American Diet (SAD) and lifestyle and become more in tune with what the body really needs to heal. To quote Dr. Clement, "Given the proper tools and environment our bodies are self-healing and self-rejuvenating".

More Natural "Cures" Revealed, by Kevin Trudeau, Alliance Publishing Group, Inc., 2006

After hearing Kevin Trudeau speak at a health conference in Chicago, my life was never the same. Ever since his book Natural Cures "They" Don't Want You to Know About, which saved countless people's lives and made the average person on the street into a more watchful and aware citizen of the world, not so blindly following doctors, Big Pharma and the FDA (just to name a few). Learning that our government is not necessarily out for what is best for us is a hard pill to swallow. In this book Kevin Trudeau hits another home run for medical freedom. He is a true "Health Freedom Warrior".

The government (not just the US either) would love to lock him up and shut him up forever. Good luck Kevin. I've joined the believers.

The Only Answer to Cancer, Defeating the Root Cause of All Disease, by Leonard Coldwell, NMD, ND, PhD., CNHP, Healing Nature Press, 2010

Instinct Based Medicine, How to Survive Your Illness and Your Doctor, Dr. Leonard Coldwell, Strategic Book Publishing, 2008

Dr. Coldwell's books take an in-depth look at the mental and environmental stress that weakens our immune systems and opens our bodies up for the onslaught of many diseases including cancer. Dr. Coldwell's success rate for treating cancer patients in his clinic in Germany is unsurpassed to date. Before his retirement and subsequent move to the U.S., he treated over 35,000 patients. His detox methods, supplement regime, and his IBMS patented therapies are discussed in detail. I listen to his CD series every night before going to sleep. Contact www.instinctbasedmedicine.com.

Sugar Blues, by William Duffy, Warner Book, Inc., 1975
This is a classic. Sugar- refined sucrose, $C12 H22 O11$, produced by multiple chemical processing of the juice of the sugar cane or beet and removal of all fiber and protein, which amount to 90 per cent of the natural plant. Sugar is one of the major ingredients in countless foods that we eat and drink, from cereal to soup, from cola to coffee. It is ingested by the hundreds of pounds by every American every year. It is as addictive as heroin and as poisonous. Refined sugar is responsible for countless illnesses ranging from depression to heart disease.

Superfoods, The Food and Medicine of the Future, by David Wolfe, North Atlantic Books, 2009
This book is simple to read, loaded with incredible information on the top 10 Superfoods from around the world. Gojo berries, cacao, maca, bee pollen, Spirulina, AFA Blue Green Algae, marine phytoplankton, aloe vera, hempseed and coconuts receive the top spot. The honorable mention foods: acai, camu camu, chlorella, Incan berries, kelp, noni and yakon are also covered quite thoroughly. His coverage of each Superfood is so in-depth it includes: geographical information, history, benefits, nutritional profile, and beautiful photographs of each Superfood. Throw in some good recipes and you've got another great book from David Wolfe.

Supplements Exposed The Truth They Don't Want You to Know About Vitamins, Minerals, and Their Effects on Your Health, Brian R. Clement, PhD, Career Press Inc., 2010
Another book by Dr. Clement that shows the incredible depth of this man's knowledge of nutrition and the many aspects of synthetic vs. whole food supplementation which is important information to know. A great resource book to take with you when you shop for vitamins.

CD Healing in the Kitchen, Raw Food Video Recipes to Transform Your Health, by Kim and David Hostetter, Raw Food Chefs
From basic sprouting to gourmet entrees and desserts this 4CD set is chock full of incredible, hands on, information on raw foods. The recipes are delicious and not too complicated. A valuable tool for everyone, particularly the vegan and novice raw food chef like me.

EPILOGUE

In my search for wellness I met wonderful, caring alternative health care providers. They treat the whole body and the mind. I've always believed that prayer changes things. Make sure your prayers (intentional or not) are positive. Forget the past and don't worry so much about the future and live for "now". It truly is all that we ever have. Forgive yourself; forgive your so-called enemies...Practice gratitude. Be grateful for every hour that you've been given. Bless everything....your food, water, vitamins, friends, family, doctors, I mean everything... and the blessings will start pouring into your own life. Feel the blessings all around you. Okay, you got sick, so does everyone at some point. So what! Get over it. Get tough! If I can do it so can you. Get going...Grab for that "brass ring." Love yourself just as you are and watch the magic start to happen in your life. Good luck, God bless you. Let's get healthy together. It really isn't that hard. Just do it.

Remember to be patient and kind to yourself. Take "baby steps"... soon you'll be walking for miles. There is an old saying "you can eat an elephant if you only take one bite at a time". Cancer is my elephant... one bite at a time until it is all gone. Go for it. You can eat your elephant if it is cancer or some other chronic diseases... remember one bite at a time. Baby steps, get up every morning and start out by being grateful that you woke up. Then, if you need to, only think "what do I have to do this hour". It gets easier and easier, trust me. Soon you'll have energy and feel good again. What miracles await you.

Look to the future. Create some goals for yourself. I challenge you to write a vision statement and a mission statement as I was challenged to do at Hippocrates Health Institute. Here is mine.

VISION STATEMENT

The journey of a thousand years begins with a single seed of inner light. Implementing the steps to create the "Greater Good Community of Mankind" to preserve our species as well as stopping the mass extinction of many others. Show the whole world the value of Enlightenment through self-education, spiritual growth through prayer, meditation and inner stillness, physical health, strength and endurance through movement of the body and thoughtful consumption of clean water, fresh air and plant based foods with inner light and Life-Force. Make an impact on the healing consciousness present in all of us by facilitating recognition of the fact that we are all one consciousness and connected energetically to each other; thereby eliminating the "I" as a separate entity and coming to seek the Greater Good for everyone. Each stone of enlightenment cast into the infinite sea of life energy will ripple forever. Change is certain. I choose to be a force for positive change.

MISSION STATEMENT

Enlighten 100,000 people by exposing them to lectures, teachers, philosophers, doctors and survivors of allopathic medical death sentences, who join me in my beliefs and vision that we need to clean up the world in order to preserve it. We will show these people the simplicity of the way: eat raw living plant based foods for nourishment; meditate for inner awareness of the power of our minds when set toward a path of positive thinking through love, joy, compassion and trust of our collective intention for seeing and creating the "Greater Good Community of Mankind"; exercise for physical strength and detoxification; rest for rebuilding the mind-body-spirit; and energy based healing tools for restoring a weakened immune system to perfect health. Four simple steps to bring us back to the One, the Creator, and the Light. Restoring balance again in all things... restoring the "Greater Good" philosophy buried somewhere in all of us.

It's great to think globally, but begin with implementing the positive things you've learned into practical terms. I will start a "Lifestyle and Nutrition Coaching" business. I call mine "Healthy Choices". It is my time to start giving back in some small way.

OBJECTIVES

1. Explain to patients that using Dr. Lubecki's protocols will heal their immune system thereby allowing their immune system to heal their bodies. With the addition of proper nutrition from a raw, living, organic, plant based diet they can create the "Lifeforce"-the perfect health that we all deserve.
2. Introduce patients, caregivers and family members to Hippocrates Protocols first with 12 DVD series. Loads of invaluable information.
3. Offer training in food preparation, juicing, sprouting, kitchen setup, all essential areas to include children as well as other family members in process.
4. Introduce meditation, yoga, Qigong. Power of positive attitude, words and thoughts.
5. Explain laser, homeopathic imprinter, and other technologies – in depth training.
6. Go over list of important books to read for more in depth study of personal interest: quantum physics, healing energy, wheatgrass, life force foods, supplementation, and environmental toxins.
7. Help patients prepare to go home with some practical tools, ideas, and websites to begin their journey to wellness now.

8. Discuss detoxification, wheatgrass implants, colonics, and lymphatic drainage.
9. Explain enzyme therapies and footbath detoxification.
10. Inspire patient and family by giving them love, joy and hope. Help them understand the power of prayer and laughter. Help them find peace, no matter what the outcome of their health challenge.

REFERENCES

Ageless Body, Timeless Mind
Deepak Chopra, Harmony Books, New York, NY

An End to Cancer?
Leon Chaitow, Thorsons Publishers Limited, Wellingborough
Northhamptonshire, England

*The Beautiful Truth: The World's Simplest Cure for
Cancer*
Steve Kroschel, CinemaLibreDistribution.com

The Biology of Belief
Bruce Lipton, Elite Books, Santa Rosa, CA

Bypassing Bypass
Elmer Cranton, M.D., and Arline Brecher, Stein and Day
Scarborough House, Briarcliff Manor, NY 10510

Cancer: A Healing Crisis
Jack Tropp, Cancer Book House, Cancer Control Society 2034
N. Berendo, Los Angeles, CA 90027

Cancer And Its Nutritional Therapies
Dr. Richard A. Passwater, Keat's Publishing, Inc., 27
Pine Street, New Canaan, CT 06840

Cancer and Vitamin C
Ewan Cameron and Linus Pauling,
The Linus Pauling Institute of Science and Medicine 2700
San Hill Road, Menlo Park, CA 94025

The Cancer Answer...Nutrition
Maureen Salaman, Stanford Publishing
1259 El Camino Real, Menlo Park, CA 94025
The Cancer Blackout
Maurice Natenrbergh, Cancer Control Society,
2043 N. Berendo, Los Angeles, CA 90027

Cancer Free – Your Guide to Gentle Non-Toxic Healing
Bill Henderson, Book Locker, Inc. 2008

The Cancer Prevention Diet
Michio Kushi, Saint Martins Press 175 5th Ave., New York, NY
10010

A Cancer Therapy, Results of Fifty Cases
Max Gerson, M.D., Totality Books
PO Box 1035, Del Mar, CA 92014

Candida, Silver (Mercury) Fillings and the Immune System
Betsy Russell Manning, Greenswood Press
1600 Larkin #104, San Francisco, CA 94109

A Challenging Second Opinion
John A. McDougall, M.D., New Century Publishers, Inc.,
220 Old New Brunswick Road, Piscatoway, NJ 08854

The Causes And Prevention Of Cancer
Dr. Frederick B. Levenson, Stein and Day, Scarborough
House, Briar Cliff Manor, NY 10510

The Chelation Answer
Morton Walker, D.P.M., M. Evans and Company, Inc., 216
East 49th Street, New York, NY 10017

The China Study, Startling Implications for Diet, Weight Loss and Long-Term Health
T. Colin Campbell and Thomas Campbell, BenBella Books, Dallas, TX 2006

Confession Of A Medical Heretic
Robert S. Mendelsohn, M.D., Warner Books, Inc., 666 Fifth Ave., New York, NY 10103

The Conquest Of Cancer
Dr. Virginia Livingston-Wheeler and Edmond G. Addeo, Franklin Watts,
387 Park Ave. South, New York, NY 10016

Counsels on Diet and Foods
Ellen G. White, Ellen G. White Publications

The Death of Cancer
Dr Harold W. Manner, Advanced Century Publishing Corp.
PO Box 1052 Evanston, IL 60204

Dental Caries As A Cause Of Nervous Disorders
Patrick Stortebecker, M.D., Ph.D., Bio-Probe, Inc., P.O. Box 58010, Orlando, FL 32858

Diet for a New America: How Your Food Choices Affect Your Health, Happiness, and the Future of Life on Earth
John Robbins, Stillpoint Publishing, Walpole, NH

Dr. Kelley's Answer To Cancer
William D. Kelly, Wedgestone Press P.O. Box 175, Winfield, KS 67156

Eating
Third Edition RaveDiet.com, Copyright 2008

The Engine 2 Diet
Rip Esselstyne, Wellness Central Publishing, 207 Park
Ave., NY, NY 10017

Enzyme Nutrition – The Food Enzyme Concept
Dr. Edward Howell, Avery Publishing Group, Inc.,
Wayne, NJ

*Fit for Life: A New Beginning – The Ultimate Diet and
Health Plan*
Harvey Diamond, Kensington Books, New York, NY

The Grape Cure
Johanna Brandt, Ehret Literature Publishing Co., Inc.,
Dobbs Ferry, NY 10522-0024

The Great Medical Monopoly Wars
P. J. Lisa, Int. Institute of Natural Health Sciences, Inc., P.O.
Box 5550, Huntington Beach, CA 92615

Healing and Recovery
David R. Hawkins, M.D., Ph.D., Veritas Publishing,
PO Box 3516, W. Sedona, AZ 86340

Healing Cancer – From The Inside Out
Mike Anderson, RaveDiet.com, 2008

Healthful Cuisine
Anna Marie Clement, Ph.D., N.M.D. with Chef Kelly
Serbonich, Healthful Communications, Inc., 13700 US
Highway One, Suite 202A, June Beach, FL 33408

Hippocrates Life Force – Superior Health and Longevity
Brian R. Clement, Ph.D., NMD, LNC, Healthy Living
Publications, Summertown, TN

How You Can Beat The Killer Diseases
Harold Harper, M.D., and Michael Culbert
Arlington House Publishers, New Rochelle, NY
Infertility & Birth Defects
Sam Ziff and Dr. Michael R. Ziff, Bio-Probe Inc., PO.
Box 58010, Orlando, FL 32858

Living Foods for Optimum Health
Brian R. Clement with Theresa Foy Digeronimo,
Three Rivers Press, New York, NY

*Living Foods for Optimum Health: Staying Healthy in an
Unhealthy World*
Brian Clement, Prima Publishing, Roseville, CA

The Macrobiotic Approach to Cancer
Michio Kushi and the East West Foundation
Avery Publishing Group, Inc., Wayne, NJ

A Documentary *Making A Killing – The Untold Story of
Psychotropic Drugging*
Citizens Commission on Human Rights

*Mercury Poisoning From Dental Amalgam - A
Hazard To The Human Brain*
Patrick Stortebecker, M.D., Ph.D., Bio-Probe, Inc., P.O.
Box 58010, Orlando, FL 32858

Naked Empress-Or The Great Medical Fraud
Hans Ruesch, Civis-Schweiz Postfach, 323 CH-
8030 Zurich, Switzerland

The Only Answer To Cancer – Defeating The Root Cause Of All Disease
Dr. Leonard Coldwell, Healing Nature Press, Springfield, MO 65807

Patient Heal Thyself
Jordan S. Rubin, N.M.D, C.N.C., Freedom Press, 1801 Chart Trail, Topanga, CA 90290

Raw Foods Bible
Craig B. Sommers, N.D., C.N., Guru Beant Press, a division of You Can Do It Productions

A Return to Love: Reflections on the Principles of A Course in Miracles
Marianne Williamson, Harper Collins Publishers, 10 Est. 53rd Street, NY, NY 10022 Publishers

Silver Dental Fillings-The Toxic Time Bomb
San Ziff, Aurora Press, 205 Third Ave. 2A, New York, NY 10003

Sprouts the Miracle Food – The Complete Guide to Sprouting
Steve Meyerowitz, Book Publishing Co., PO Box 99, Summertown, TN 38483

Survival in the 21st Century – Planetary Healers Manual
Viktoras H. Kulvinskas, M.S. Book Publishing Co., Summertown, TN

The Wheatgrass Book
Ann Wigmore, Avery Publishing Group, Inc., Wayne, NJ

Wheatgrass – Nature's Finest Medicine
Steve Meyerowitz, Book Publishing Co., PO Box 99,
Summertwon, TN 38483

World Without Cancer
G. Edward Griffin, American Media,
PO Box 4646, Westlake Village, CA *91359*

The Yeast Connection
William G. Crook, M.D., Professional Books, P.O.
Box 3494, Jackson, TN 38301

The Yeast Syndrome
John Parks Trowbridge, M.D., and Morton Walker, D.P.M.,
Bantam Books, Inc., 666 Fifth Ave., New York, NY 10103

CPSIA information can be obtained at www.ICGtesting.com
Printed in the USA
LVOW081548051112

305902LV00002B/155/P